Intermittent Fasting for Women Over 50

The Essential Guide to Lose Weight,
Detox Your Body, Boost Your Energy
and Brain Function.
Healthy Recipes and 35-Day Meal Plan
Included

Mary K. Day

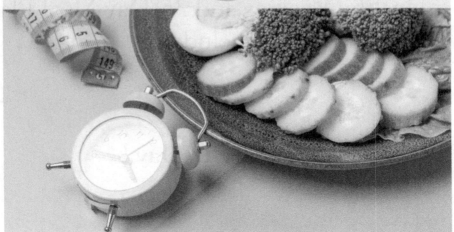

Table of Contents

Introduction

Fasting has been known for its physical and mental benefits since ancient times. It was described by Plato and Aristotle and is part of the rituals of many religions.

Recent scientific studies have proven what the ancients always said: fasting is a healthy cure-all. In particular, fasting has been shown to offer several benefits for women after 50. In fact, usually at this stage of life, women undergo significant hormonal changes and go through menopause and related problems.

I have seen many women struggle with weight gain during menopause, which can be difficult. But don't worry; Intermittent Fasting is here to help.

In this book, you'll discover how Intermittent Fasting works and how it can help you cope with menopause problems to stay young and in great shape. While a conventional diet focuses on what to eat, Intermittent Fasting concentrates mainly on when. In this eating strategy, you alternate between extreme or complete restriction of calories (fasting) and periods of healthy eating. Depending on personal choice, the duration of these calorie-restricted and healthy-eating cycles varies.

We'll explore in the simplest way possible the science behind Intermittent Fasting and why it works, especially for women over 50. We will delve into the different benefits of Intermittent Fasting, such as weight loss, reduced inflammation, and improved brain function.

After a detailed overview of the different Intermittent Fasting protocols, I will guide you in choosing the best for your needs.

You'll get practical advice on how to start your Intermittent Fasting journey. I'll help you prepare your mind, set your goals, organize your pantry, and measure your success.

Not all people mention that Intermittent Fasting has challenges, such as hunger pains, digestive problems, cravings, headaches, weakness, sleep disturbances, and dehydration. We'll go through them all and see some strategies for solving them.

We'll also dispel the false myths about Intermittent Fasting, answering all the questions and doubts that usually arise for those beginning to venture into this lifestyle.

In the last part of the book, I will also provide you with healthy and easy recipes for breakfast, main dishes, snacks, and smoothies to make your fasting journey enjoyable and delicious. Finally, you will find a special BONUS: a 35-day meal plan for women over 50, with different daily options to master your new stress-free eating habits.

Intermittent Fasting can be a game changer for shedding weight by successfully embracing a healthy lifestyle full of new energy. With this book, you will have all the information you need and get the most out of your Intermittent Fasting journey. Let's get started!

Chapter 1: Intermittent Fasting for Women Over 50 Overview

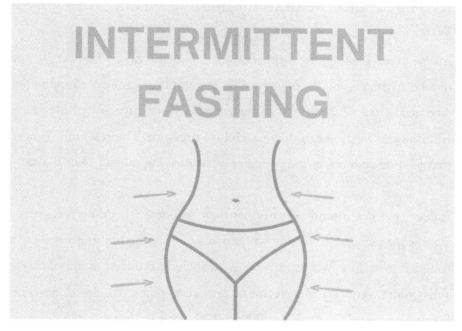

We all know losing weight can be difficult for women over 50. A variety of factors can cause this difficulty. The most common cause is a slow metabolism. The faster the metabolism, the more fat we eliminate. However, as we grow older, we lose lean muscle mass, and we tend to accumulate fat. In addition, we become less active than we used to be. What is the end result? Stubborn body fat that refuses to go away.

Intermittent Fasting has grown in popularity in recent years due to its many health benefits and the fact that it does not restrict meal choices. According to some research, Fasting has been shown to increase mental health, speed up metabolism and possibly prevent several malignancies.

It may also protect women over 50 from specific muscle, nerve, and joint diseases.

1.1 The Science Behind Intermittent Fasting And Why It Works

Intermittent Fasting for women over 50 might help lose weight and reduce the possibility of typically developing age-related ailments. According to a new research study by the Baylor University of Medicine, Intermittent Fasting can decrease blood pressure. The research showed that Fasting reduces blood pressure by improving the gut microbiota.

Indeed, besides intending to boost their wellness, shedding weight is a significant concern for many women over 50. Some points that make it tougher to reduce weight after age 50 include reduced metabolic rate, achy joints, reduced muscle mass, and rest issues. At the same time, losing fat, especially unsafe stubborn belly fat can dramatically decrease your threat of such severe health issues as diabetic issues, cardiovascular disease, and cancer cells.

The risk of developing many conditions rises as you age. In some cases, periodic Fasting for females over 50 might serve as a stream of youth when it involves weight reduction and reduces the opportunity to develop commonly age-related health problems. At its most basic level, intermittent Fasting merely aids the body in utilizing its surplus resources by digesting excess body fat. It's essential to remember that this is a natural phenomenon, and humans have evolved by fasting for short periods - days or hours — without suffering significant health consequences. Body fat is generally accumulated as a result of an excess of calories. If you don't eat, your body will "consume" its fat for sustenance. It's all about finding the correct balance in life—the good and the terrible, the yin and the yang. The same may be said of food and abstention. Fasting is, in general, the polar opposite of eating. When they don't eat, they are fasting. It works as follows:

We supply more nutritional calories when we feed more than we need. Any remaining fuel is put aside for later use. Insulin is a hormone that aids in storing energy obtained from the diet. Our insulin levels rise when we eat, which helps us keep more energy in two ways. Carbs are essential food nutrients broken down into glucose units that can be combined to form glycogen and stored within the liver or muscle.

On the other hand, Sugars have a finite storage capacity, and once that limit is reached, the liver starts to convert the excess glucose to fat. This process is called de-novo lipogenesis ("creating new fat"). Although some of the newly generated fat is stored in the liver, most are transported to other fatty tissue throughout the body. Even though this is a more complex operation, the amount of fat that can be made is nearly endless.

There are two major energy storage systems in the human body. One is easy to use but has limited storage capacity (glycogen), while another is more difficult to utilize but has practically unlimited storage capacity (glucose) (lipids). The mechanism reverses if we do not feed. Because food is no longer available, insulin levels drop, signaling the body to utilize stored energy. Because blood sugar levels are declining, the liver must pull glucose from its reserves to power itself. The most readily available energy source is glucose. It is degraded into sugar molecules to deliver sugar to the body's other cells. This will continue for 24-36 hours and provide enough energy to meet most of the body's requirements. A fat breakdown would then become the body's principal source of nutrition. As a result, the body can only exist in two states: fed or fasted.

We are either expanding food storage or depleting stored energy (burning stored energy) (decreasing stores). It's a choice between these two options. There can be no net weight difference if feeding and abstinence are equal. Whether we start feeding as soon as we get out of bed and don't stop until we sleep, we waste roughly half of our lives in the fed state. Over time, we may gain weight if we do not provide our bodies with enough energy to burn stored dietary fuel. To regain equilibrium or lose weight, we need to increase the time we spend utilizing energy from food. It's known as intermittent Fasting.

Intermittent Fasting, however, allows the body to use any residual fat. It's important to remember that there's nothing wrong with it. That is how our bodies are created. Dogs, mice, bears, and wolves all do this. That is exactly what women do. If you feed every two hours, your body can always use the new food resources as is commonly recommended. It may not be sufficient to burn off much if any, body fat. You may be just gaining weight. Your body is likely storing it for a day when you won't be able to feed yourself. You will be out of control if this happens. Intermittent Fasting is something you need to catch up on.

Fasting affects most hormones in the body, including the appetite hormones ghrelin and leptin. As previously stated, intermittent Fasting lowers ghrelin levels and can promote weight loss. Intermittent Fasting may aid weight loss by lowering blood glucose and insulin levels and lowering LDL ("bad") cholesterol, triglyceride levels, and inflammation. However, it's worth mentioning that most studies on how intermittent Fasting affects body chemistry have been conducted on men.

1. The Problem With The Modern Age: Feeding Vs. Fasting

Humans did not evolve to eat multiple small meals throughout the day and nighttime. On the other hand, humans also adapted to daily fasts: we survived hunting and gathering until the birth of agriculture some 12,000 years ago, and we did it mainly with hungry bellies. Regularly, we are designed to undertake Intermittent Fasting. Furthermore, women eat during times of the day when they could have previously slept. Because late-night television and other electrically powered entertainments (such as Zoom sessions) drive us to sit up late and nibble late, our evening fasting phase began much earlier than it does now for millennia.

First, understanding how Intermittent Fasting helps women lose weight is essential to understand the difference between fed and fasted states. The body is in a fed state when it digests and absorbs food. The fed state starts when you start feeding and lasts 3 to 5 hours as your body digests and absorbs the nutrition you just ate. It is tough for your body to burn fat while in the fed state since your insulin levels are elevated.

During that time, the body enters a condition known as the post-absorptive condition, which is just a refined way of saying that it isn't digesting the food. Before you enter the fasted state, you are still in the post-absorptive stage, 8 to 12 hours after your last meal. It is considerably easier for your body to lose fat while fasting because your insulin levels are low.

Fasting permits the body to digest previously inaccessible fat, primarily while eating. Our bodies are rarely in this fat-burning state if we haven't fasted for more than 12 hours after our previous meal. This is one of the main reasons many women who start Intermittent Fasting lose weight without changing their diet, food intake, or activity frequency. Fasting causes your body to enter a fat-burning state difficult to reach with a regular eating schedule.

2. Menopause And Weight Gain: What Science Says

Menopause is a challenging period in a woman's life. You devote nearly every waking hour to the gym. You only eat chicken breasts, fish, and vegetables. On the other hand, the numbers on the scale refuse to compromise — or, more likely, they're progressively increasing along with your waist circumference. What is it about menopause that leads you to gain weight and makes it much more difficult to lose weight? It's almost certainly a mix of menopausal and aging-related factors. As a result of the transition, many women experience changes, such as weight gain that defies all attempts to reverse it. Women frequently assume that they are to blame regarding their weight.

On the other hand, hormonal fluctuations and other menopause-related changes are often to blame. These have no bearing on what they're doing. Understanding why women acquire weight during menopause might help them accept this natural occurrence and better manage their weight in the future to support their health. As a woman in her mid-to-late 40s, you may notice that your favorite blue mom jeans are becoming noticeably tighter, aside from the occasional flare-up or poor mood. This time it's not in your head. According to classic research, when a woman reaches menopause in her 40s, she gains roughly four and a half pounds. A recent study issued in the Mayo Clinic journal states that it's also a trend that doesn't seem to be slowing down: Women in their 50s and 60s continue to gain around a pound and a half per year. The leading cause is natural skeletal muscle loss as women age. When muscle consumes more calories than fat, your metabolism slows, allowing you to gain weight. According to scientists, starting at 30, you lose around a half-pound of muscle per year, which grows to about a full pound by age 50.

As you move through menopause, you may notice the following: Even if the number on the chart doesn't appear to be increasing much, whatever extra weight you gain tends to accumulate all over your stomach, leaving you a fat belly. During menopause, your ovaries stop producing estrogen; it may only be created in your belly fat tissue. As a result, the body naturally gravitates toward fat storage in that location to receive estrogen. Experts have dubbed the stomach "the third ovary." This type of fat, which is named visceral fat, is, nevertheless, dangerous. It produces stress hormones such as cortisol, as well as damaging cytokines. These substances induce your body to create more insulin, resulting in an increase in fat storage in fat cells and an increase in appetite. As a result, you'll gain more belly fat than ever, and you'll be more likely to develop insulin resistance, a crucial risk factor for heart failure and type 2 diabetes.

Gynoid body fat is a phenomenon in which women's butts and thighs appear to gain weight over the years. Hormone variations cause many female bodies to store excess weight around the middle during early menopause rather than after menopause, a process known as android fat distribution. It irritates women greatly. Not only are they dealing with heat sweats and other hormonal changes, but they're also dealing with a significant change in body shape. When you acquire weight around your waist, it's not just about your appearance. It's a potential health risk linked to an increased risk of medical problems like heart disease, stroke, and diabetes. This fluctuating additional weight after menopause is thought to contribute to women's higher risk of heart disease.

In animal studies, estrogen has been shown to manage body mass better. Reduced hormone levels in lab mice cause them to overeat and become less fit and healthy. Decreased estrogen can cause the body's metabolic rate or the pace it converts stored energy into usable energy to reduce. The same phenomenon probably happens to women after estrogen levels drop after menopause. According to some research, estrogen replacement medication increases a woman's basal metabolic rate. This will help you gain weight more slowly. Furthermore, estrogen deficiency can cause the body to use carbs and sugar levels inefficiently, resulting in fat buildup and making weight loss more difficult.

Other aging factors come into play as well. When women reach adulthood, they undergo several additional changes, contributing to obesity. For example, they are less likely to exercise. One-fifth of the population is insufficiently active, and this percentage climbs with age. Furthermore, our muscle mass reduces as we age, lowering our basal metabolism and making it easier to gain weight, especially for women over 50. When you exercise, the rate at which you can expend energy slows down. Regardless of your prior activity levels, if you desire to lose weight using the same amount of resources as previously, you may need to increase the length of time and strength with which you exercise.

3. What Are Men's And Women's Reactions To Intermittent Fasting?

Intermittent Fasting has many potential benefits, ranging from weight loss to longer life expectancy. Recent research suggests that female fasts have different advantages and drawbacks than males. Women are more sensitive to the effects of abstinence than men. A metabolic pathway is activated during Fasting. When this occurs, you burn fat instead of carbs for energy (or blood glucose). This could account for any of the benefits of various fasting practices. According to studies, women change faster than men when following an Intermittent fasting routine. Researchers discovered that when men and women fasted for the same amount of time, women had more fat in their circulation. Women can benefit from shorter fasting times as a result of this. For women, a 16:8 schedule may be more beneficial than an 18:6 schedule, which entails abstinence for 18 hours and eating within six hours. According to animal research, females can benefit from much shorter fasting periods than males.

Women's fat loss results have been connected to strict diets and Fasting. Most Intermittent fasts have no restrictions on what you can eat or drink during your feeding times or days. According to a study published in a journal in 2019, obese women who fasted intermittently and followed a rigorous diet lost more weight.

The age of a woman can also affect how her body reacts to skipping breakfast. According to experts, Fasting can lead postmenopausal women to shed twice as much fat as younger, premenopausal women. According to one study, postmenopausal women lost up to 24 pounds by fasting on alternate days for a year. Following a 90-day time-restricted diet, postmenopausal women shed nine pounds (also regarded as 16:8).

The truth is that everyone, not just men and women, reacts differently to Fasting. In reality, males and females have varied reactions to Intermittent Fasting. Gonadotropin-releasing hormone, which is contained in everyone, causes the gonads to react. It causes women's ovaries to create progesterone and men's testes to produce testosterone. The mechanism is closely monitored in women since it is linked to the menstrual cycle and depends on rhythms and patterns. Improved habits and routines are likely to halt gonadotropin release hormone more quickly in women than in men, but missing a meal can also cause more discomfort in women than in men. Kisspeptin, a protein that causes enhanced fasting vulnerability, was shown to be higher in females. This is merely one possibility that has to be tested further. On the other hand,

Fasting has been demonstrated in multiple rodent studies to have a negative impact on female sex hormones. Also, some human evidence suggests that women have difficulty controlling their appetite during fasts.

Fasting made men more parasympathetic, meaning a less aggravated stress response, whereas fasting made women more reactive, implying their systems were tenser, more in the "fight-or-flight" mode.

You may become more sensitive to its effects because you aren't producing as much insulin during abstinence (becoming less "insulin resistant"). Because insulin improves food digestion and carbohydrate metabolism, many consider insulin sensitivity crucial for weight loss. According to some research, alternate-day Fasting affects men and women differently. It mainly reduces glucose tolerance, connected to insulin sensitivity, in men but not women.

According to one study, when males fast for a short period, their metabolic rate improves by up to 14%. Furthermore, according to other research, the male body boosts testosterone and HGH production. These metabolic changes are necessary for tight muscles and lower disease risk. According to another study, Intermittent Fasting increased insulin responsiveness in males, but it did not affect female participants.

In actuality, women's sugar tolerance has declined. Other research on the effect of Intermittent Fasting on blood lipids found that men's "good" cholesterol remained stable as their lipids decreased. Still, women's "good" cholesterol increased while their lipids remained stable.

1.2 Different Benefits Of Intermittent Fasting

Several studies have demonstrated Intermittent Fasting offers significant mental and physical health benefits. When you begin fasting, you will experience the following advantages:

Let's have a look at how Intermittent Fasting can help you lose weight effortlessly, regulate your hormones, strengthen your immune system, reduce inflammation, manage menopause, help you delay aging, keep and improve your physical appearance and body tone, increase energy, boost your brain functions, improve mood, control anxiety, and depression[1].

1. How Intermittent Fasting Can Help You Lose Weight

There are three main reasons why Intermittent Fasting helps you lose weight:

1)by reducing your eating time, you reduce your calorie intake. Taking in fewer calories helps prevent your body from accumulating nutrients it doesn't need that would be stored as fat;

2)it regulates hunger hormones, drastically reducing the chance that you will indulge in unnecessary snacks during eating time;

3)it speeds up your metabolism and reduces your insulin levels, which helps your body burn stored fat.

According to a 2014 review, Intermittent Fasting decreased body weight by 3–8% over just 3–24 weeks.

Regarding weight loss, Intermittent Fasting could generate weight loss of 0.55 to 1.65 pounds (0.25–0.75 kg) every week.

The participants' waist circumference decreased by 3–7%, indicating that they lost belly fat.

Collier R. Intermittent fasting: the science of going without. CMAJ. 2013 Jun 11;185(9):E363-4. doi: 10.1503/cmaj.109-4451. Epub 2013 Apr 8. PMID: 23569168; PMCID: PMC3680567.[1]

These results suggest that Intermittent Fasting could be an extremely effective strategy for losing weight.

However, the advantages of Intermittent Fasting go far beyond weight loss.

It also has a range of metabolic health benefits and can help reduce the risk level of cardiovascular disease.

Calorie counting is not mandatory when fasting; weight loss is primarily mediated by reducing overall calorie consumption.

Studies comparing Intermittent Fasting with continuous calorie restriction indicate no difference in weight loss whenever the groups match calories.

Intermittent Fasting is a simple technique to shed pounds without having to control calories. Many studies have shown that it can aid in weight loss and reduce abdominal fat.

2. How Intermittent Fasting Regulates Your Hormones

When you don't eat for quite a while, your body goes through several changes.

Your body, for example, alters hormone levels to make the stored body fat more accessible while initiating critical cellular repair processes.

There are some of the physiological changes that occur during Fasting:

- **Insulin levels are high.** Insulin levels in the blood drop, allowing fat to be burned more efficiently.

- **Levels of human growth hormone (HGH).** Human growth hormone levels in the blood could skyrocket. Increased levels of this hormone help with fat loss and muscle gain, among other things.

- **Repairing cellular structures**. The body induces important cellular repair activities - such as removing waste material from cells.

- **Expression of genes.** Several genes and substances linked to longevity and illness resistance have undergone favorable modifications.

These changes in hormones, cell function, and gene expression are linked to many advantages of Intermittent Fasting.

Insulin levels decline, and human growth hormone (HGH) levels rise when you fast. Your cells also launch critical cellular repair processes and alter the expression of genes.

3. How Intermittent Fasting Strengthens Your Immune System

According to a University of Southern California research, prolonged Fasting can lead to immune system cell regeneration.

When we first start fasting, our bodies break down many immune-fighting white blood cells. It automatically recognizes the need to conserve energy, and one way it does so is by eliminating old or damaged immune cells. However, it swiftly adapts and initiates the regeneration of new cells, increasing the number of immune-boosting cells in our bodies.

This discovery prompted extensive research into Intermittent Fasting, defined as a fast lasting 16 hours or longer each day. According to a study, when we stop eating because the food content is low, cells in the body that promote the immune response and battle invading pathogens leave the bloodstream. They travel to nutrient-dense bone marrow, where they rebuild and become supercharged, better protecting the body from infection.

4. How Intermittent Fasting Can Help Reduce The Body Inflammation

Intermittent Fasting, according to studies, can lower inflammation in the body.

Inflammation is one of the body's defense mechanisms against infection, but too much inflammation can lead to various disorders.

According to experts, many women have an overabundance of inflammation due to eating too much and too frequently.

Our bodies release inflammatory molecules when we eat in response to the digesting process. By reducing the amount of time we spend digesting food, Intermittent Fasting can help decrease the release of these substances. Moreover, this decrease in inflammation may also depend on Intermittent Fasting's ability to lower oxidative stress and enhance cellular metabolism, which are inflammation factors.

Also, it has been demonstrated that Intermittent Fasting lowers several inflammatory biomarkers in the body, including C-reactive protein (CRP), interleukin-6 (IL-6), and tumor necrosis factor-alpha (TNF-alpha)[2].

For these reasons, Intermittent Fasting is a valuable aid in the battle against inflammation, another major cause of many diseases.

5. How Intermittent Fasting Helps Manage Menopause

Weight increase in women over 50 is prevalent, while the specific reason and effect are still being debated. Lower estrogen levels can lead to a slower metabolic rate, leading to weight gain even if we don't change our diet. Because of our increasing insulin resistance, we will be less able to metabolize carbs and sugars. Or it could be those two fat-storing and fat-synthesis enzymes, which are much more active in postmenopausal women, causing menopause weight increase. It could be the decreased muscular mass, which causes us to burn fewer calories even when resting. Unfortunately, many women have a rise in ghrelin, the hunger hormone, and a decrease in leptin, which signals when we're full[3].

Intermittent Fasting can handle a variety of menopausal symptoms, including:

[2] Feng, V., Bawa, K., Marzolini, S., Kiss, A., Oh, P., Herrmann, N., Lanctôt, K., & Gallagher, D. (2021). Impact of 12-week exercise program on biomarkers of gut barrier integrity in patients with coronary artery disease. PLoS One, 16(11), e0260165.
[3] Novak, J., & Gillis, B. (2022). A primer on sleep for MFTs: Implications and practical considerations. Journal of Marital and Family Therapy, 48(2), 543.

- **Gaining weight.** Intermittent Fasting has been shown to aid fat loss in studies, so many women find it an excellent long-term approach for keeping small.

- **Insulin resistance.** This is the condition in which Fasting improves insulin sensitivity, allowing your body to handle sugar and carbohydrates more efficiently. It may also reduce your chances of a heart attack, diabetes, or other metabolic problems.

- **Changes in mental health.** Anxiety, despair, exhaustion, brain fog, mood fluctuations, and psychological stress are common symptoms of menopause. Studies have shown fasting boosts self-esteem, reduces depression and anxiety, and promotes good psychological changes.

- **Brain Fog.** According to animal studies, fasting shields brain cells from stress, helping them clear out waste products, repair themselves, and make them more efficient. There hasn't been any research on how Fasting impacts the human brain, yet greater mental clarity is one of the most common paired effects. Although the data for this advantage isn't conclusive, you can try fasting and see whether you notice a difference.

6. How Intermittent Fasting Can Help You Delay Aging

There's no doubt that having youthful, radiant skin makes you appear more attractive. Nothing sparkles brighter than healthy, glowing skin, no matter how pricey the treatments and cosmetics are. All we need to look beautiful is a healthy body and a clear mind.

However, we frequently overlook our health, and our appearance merely reflects our inside wellness. We are what we eat, and our skin mirrors our health, revealing whatever we feed it!

Our metabolism is the cornerstone of a healthy and youthful complexion, but what occurs when we start intermittent Fasting? Does this affect your skin and cause it to age?

Fasting can assist the body in keeping a healthy balance to some extent, but going on an extended and austere fast to lose weight can harm your general health, with noticeable evidence on the skin.

As per a recent study, Fasting boosts the body's metabolic activity, resulting in a healthier body and skin. Furthermore, it has anti-aging properties. In fact, fad diets such as intermittent Fasting can help women over 50 lose weight and live longer.

Dr. Takayuki Teruya and a team of experts from the Okinawa Institute of Science and Technology Graduate University in Japan studied the impact of metabolism on skin aging. Fasting and calorie restriction increase metabolism and immunity, according to a study.

7. How Intermittent Fasting Can Improve Your Physical Appearance And Body Tone

Weight loss and detoxification are two benefits of Intermittent Fasting that improve your physical appearance and tone up your body. Weight loss occurs because the body burns carbs first. Indeed, if the carbs are not replaced, the body turns to fat for energy.

Intermittent Fasting detoxifies the body. All toxins in your body are eliminated during detoxification, leaving you with better skin and much less bloating.

Dieting has the unfortunate adverse effect of causing muscle and fat loss. In specific trials, intermittent Fasting has proven effective for preserving muscle mass while reducing body fat.

According to a scholarly review, intermittent calorie restriction led to a comparable degree of weight loss as constant calorie restriction but with a significantly lower decrease in muscle mass.

In the calorie-restricted studies, muscle mass lost 25% of the weight loss, compared to 10% in the intermittent calorie-restricted studies.

These studies, however, have some flaws, so take the results with a pinch of salt. Recent studies have indicated no differences in lean mass or muscle mass during Intermittent Fasting compared to other eating patterns.

8. How Can Intermittent Fasting Boost Your Brain Functions, Improve Mood, Control Anxiety And Depression

Intermittent Fasting boosts the production of a neurotropic factor generated from the brain (BDNF).

Higher levels of BDNF have been shown to improve psychological and mental performance. This particular kind of protein interacts with other brain regions to regulate cognition, learning, and cognitive functions.

The neurotrophic factor derived from the brain can also protect and improve the connections between neurons.

The brain hormone BDNF is increased when you fast. It's plausible that it's the origin of new brain cell growth. In multiple investigations, Intermittent Fasting has been demonstrated to help treat Alzheimer's disease. Intermittent Fasting boosts brain capacity while also improving cognitive functions. Intermittent Fasting causes the body to enter a ketogenic state, in which ketones are being used to convert excess weight to fuel. Ketones will also provide energy to the brain, improving cognitive efficiency, endurance, and alertness.

Intermittent Fasting activates a process known as autophagy, during which your brain "cleans up" the garbage it accumulates throughout the day. This self-cleaning mechanism promotes the detoxification of the brain and the removal of old and damaged cells and residue. This nocturnal cleaning aids the regeneration of fresher, healthier cells. Autophagy dysfunction has been related to Alzheimer's disease, depression, schizophrenia, bipolar disorder, and other neuropsychiatric illnesses.

According to a study published in the Journal of Nutrition Health and Aging, research participants reported improved moods and less tension, irritability, and disorientation after three months of Intermittent Fasting. It was linked to considerable gains in emotional well-being and sadness, according to a 2018 study looking into weight-loss regimens.

Chapter 2: Intermittent Fasting Protocols for Women Over 50

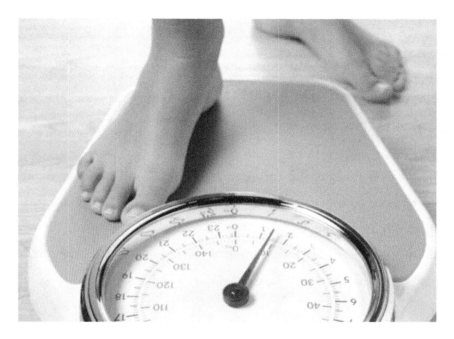

There are multiple approaches to practicing Intermittent Fasting. Among the most popular are:

- the 16:8 method

- Eat Stop Eat

- the 5:2 diet

- the Warrior diet

- Alternate-Day Fasting (ADF)

- OMAD (one meal a day)

All strategies can be helpful, but determining which works best for you is a personal decision.

Here's a rundown of the benefits and drawbacks of each strategy to help you decide which is best for you.

2.1 The 16/8 Method

One of the most popular weight-loss fasting plans is the 16/8 Intermittent Fasting strategy.

The method restricts the consumption of food and calorie-containing beverages to an 8-hour time window per day. It requires fasting for the other 16 hours of the day.

While other diets may have stringent restrictions and regulations, the 16/8 technique is more flexible and is based on the time-restricted feeding (TRF) concept.

You can consume calories over any 8 hours.

Some women avoid eating late and stick to a 9 a.m. to 5 p.m. routine, while others skip breakfast and fast from midday to 8 p.m.

Limiting the number of hours, you can eat throughout the day may aid in weight loss and blood pressure reduction.

According to research, time-restricted meal patterns, such as the 16/8 approach, can help avoid hypertension and minimize food consumption, resulting in weight loss.

In a 2016 study, the 16/8 approach effectively reduced fat mass and retained muscle mass in the male participants when paired with resistance training.

A recent study discovered that the 16/8 method did not affect muscle or strength gains in resistance training women.

While the 16/8 approach can be readily incorporated into any lifestyle, some women may struggle to go 16 hours without eating.

Furthermore, consuming too many snacks or junk food throughout your 8-hour fasting window can counteract the benefits of 16/8 Intermittent Fasting.

To reap the most health benefits from this diet, consume a well-balanced diet rich in fruits, vegetables, healthy fats, whole grains, and protein.

2.2 Eat-Stop-Eat

The author Brad Pilon popularized an innovative technique for Intermittent Fasting called "Eat Stop Eat."[4]

This Intermittent Fasting method entails deciding on one or two non-consecutive days every week when you will go without eating for 24 hours.

You can eat as much as you like the rest of the week, but it's best to eat a well-balanced diet and avoid overindulging.

---

[4] Pilon, B. (2017). *Eat Stop Eat: Intermittent Fasting for Health and Weight Loss.* Self-Published.

A weekly 24-hour fast is justified by the belief that eating fewer calories will result in weight loss.

Engaging in fasting for a duration of up to 24 hours can induce a metabolic shift, prompting your body to utilize fat rather than glucose as its primary source of energy.

However, abstaining from food 24 hours a day requires significant discipline and may potentially lead to episodes of binge eating and overconsumption at a later time. It could also result in disturbed eating habits.

More research is needed to establish the Eat Stop Eat diet's possible health advantages and weight loss qualities.

Before you attempt Eat Stop Eat or any Intermittent Fasting technique, please consult a doctor to determine whether it's a reasonable weight-loss plan.

2.3 The 5:2 Method

The 5:2 diet is an easy Intermittent Fasting plan.

You can normally eat five days a week and not count calories. Next, you cut your calorie consumption to one-quarter on the remaining two days of the week.

For a person who takes in 2,000 calories daily, this would cut their calorie intake to 500 calories twice a week.

According to a report published in 2018, the 5:2 diet is just as efficient for weight loss and blood glucose control as daily calorie restriction in type 2 diabetes patients.

Another study indicated that the 5:2 diet is equally effective for weight loss and preventing metabolic disorders like heart disease and diabetes, as well as non-stop calorie moderation.

With the 5:2 diet, you may choose which days you want to fast, and you don't plan any restrictions on what or when you eat on non-fasting days. However, eating "normally" on full-calorie days doesn't really mean that you may eat anything you want.

Whether it's only for two days a week, limiting yourself to 500 calories per day is difficult. Also, eating too few calories could make you feel unwell or fain.

While the 5:2 diet can be beneficial, it is not absolutely for everyone.

Even for the 5:2 method, it is essential to consult your doctor to see if it is suitable for you, especially if you have health problems.

2.4 Alternate Day Fasting

Alternate-day Fasting is another easy-to-follow intermittent fasting plan. On this regimen, you must fast every other day but can eat what you want on non-fasting days.

Some versions of this diet follow a fasting technique that involves eating roughly 500 calories on fasting days. Other variants, on the other hand, exclude calories entirely on fasting days.

Fasting on alternate days has been shown to help women lose weight.

Research has demonstrated that alternate-day fasting is equally effective for weight loss when compared to daily calorie restriction.

Another study indicated that after alternating between 36 hours of Fasting and 12 hours of unrestrained eating for four weeks, individuals consumed 35% fewer calories and lost 7.7 pounds (3.5 kg).

If you're serious about losing weight, incorporating an exercise routine into your daily routine can assist.

According to research, mixing alternate-day Fasting with endurance exercise can result in weight loss that is twice as effective as simply fasting.

Fasting for a full day every other day might be challenging, especially if you're new to the practice. On non-fasting days, it's easy to go overboard. If you're new to intermittent Fasting, start with a modified fasting plan to ease into alternate-day Fasting.

It's ideal for maintaining a balanced diet containing high-protein foods and low-calorie veggies to help you feel full, whether you start with a reduced fasting plan or a total fast.

2.5 OMAD (One Meal a Day)

The Intermittent Fasting OMAD-one meal-a-day- diet is a plan in which you don't eat for 23 hours a day and consume all of the daily calories in one hour (within the same 4-hour window every day).

The number of calories consumed throughout the 1-hour meal session is unrestricted.

The OMAD diet can assist you in losing weight, but doctors believe the lifestyle isn't sustainable, and the diet can involve risks.

According to Dena Champion, RD, of The Ohio State University Wexner Medical Center,

OMAD could be described as "Intermittent Fasting on steroids."

"OMAD is when someone eats one meal every day for one hour and then fasts for the remaining 23 hours."

During Fasting, you may sip black coffee or other low-calorie beverages but nothing else.

Plus, according to Jen Oikarinen, a clinical dietician at Banner University Medical Center Phoenix, you should consume that one meal daily throughout the same four-hour window. "The OMAD diet emphasizes consistency," she says. While eating healthy foods is essential, Champion points out it is more about when than what you consume.

According to Oikarinen, OMAD dieters must follow a series of rules described as the "four ones rule." So, if you're following the OMAD diet, here's what you should do:

- Each day, you should consume only one meal.
- Only eat within one hour of the end of your four-hour eating window.
- You must eat a single plate.
- If you desire a calorie-containing beverage, you must limit yourself to one.

While the OMAD diet is essentially a fasting diet, it differs from the other Intermittent Fasting programs, such as the 16:8 diet, which calls for you to fast for 16 hours and then eat three (or four!) meals for the remaining eight hours.

While many people praise the OMAD diet online, some professionals do not support this form of Intermittent Fasting. Some nutritionists say that even healthy women should avoid the diet, especially pregnant women recovering from past disordered eating, breastfeeding, diabetes, or even exercising or lifting weights regularly.

"Healthy weight loss will indeed be whatever is most long-term maintainable," she explains. This includes following a nutritious diet and engaging in regular physical exercise.

Certain population groups should also avoid the OMAD diet, such as older adults, kids, and those with health disorders or who take medication. Not eating enough calories regularly can lead to significant health problems.

2.6 The Warrior Diet

The Warrior Diet is an Intermittent Fasting method that takes inspiration from the eating habits of ancient warriors.

Ori Hofmekler developed it in 2001, and it is more intense than the 16:8 techniques but less stringent than the Eat Fast and Eat method.

It involves eating relatively little during the day for 20 hours and then eating as much as wanted in a 4-hour window at night.

During the 20-hour fast, the Warrior Diet lets you eat small amounts of vegetables, raw fruits, dairy products, hard-boiled eggs, and non-calorie drinks.

Women can eat whatever they want during the 4-hour window after a 20-hour fast. You shall prefer unprocessed, healthy, and organic meals.

There are no specific studies on the Warrior Diet, but time-restricted meal cycles can result in weight loss.

In mice, time-restricted feeding cycles have been demonstrated to prevent diabetes, delay aging, decrease tumor progression, and extend life expectancy.

Further research should be done to accurately comprehend the advantages of the warrior diet for weight loss.

The Warrior Diet could be hard to stick to because it limits food consumption to only 4 hours daily. If you're up for the task, consult your physician to discover if it's suitable and safe for your needs.

Chapter 3: Practical Advice for Beginning Your Intermittent Fasting Journey

It should be clear that intermittent Fasting is not a diet in the traditional sense but a method where eating is timed. Unlike a dietary plan restricting where calories originate, intermittent Fasting does not define which foods you must eat or avoid. Although intermittent Fasting has several health benefits, notably weight loss, it is still not for everyone.

Intermittent Fasting involves alternating between eating and fasting times. Women may actually find it highly challenging at an early stage to eat only for shorter periods each day or to alternate between the eating and Fasting days. In this chapter, you'll find directions on how to get started with Fasting, including setting personal goals, preparing meals, and determining caloric requirements. Intermittent Fasting is a popular approach for achieving the following objectives:

- make your life easier
- lose weight
- minimize the consequences of aging
- increase your general health and well-being.

Fasting is generally safe for most healthy and well-nourished women. However, it may not be acceptable for those with medical issues. The following guidelines are intended to assist women ready to begin fasting in making it as simple and successful as possible.

3.1 Prepare Your Mind

Intermittent Fasting can be physically and mentally demanding. You can have days when you feel defeated because you didn't stick to your diet plan in the letter. You may become discouraged when you don't see any visible changes in your weight. It is absolutely normal. Getting down on yourself can happen, but it is a moment you can overcome.

Please remember that intermittent Fasting is a path that takes time to complete and requires ongoing mental renewal. To stay dedicated to the process, make sure you're in a healthy mental state before you start.

3.2 Determine Your Objectives

The very first step is to identify and understand your objectives. What motivates you to begin intermittent Fasting? It may have been recommended to you by a dietician or doctor for weight loss to feel more focused, break sugar cravings, or lose weight. Keep that goal in mind, whatever it is. It will assist you in deciding how to fast and which fasting strategy to try.

Calculate and track your macros if you want to reduce weight or gain muscle. Because your feeding window will be smaller than usual, you'll need to know how many calories and nutrients you need to meet your objectives.

3.3 Prepare Your Pantry

Planning your meals and filling your pantry with the right foods to achieve your goal will be very helpful when you start caring for your nutrition.

Meal preparation does not have to be limiting. It considers calorie intake and ensures that the diet includes the proper nutrients.

Meal planning has many advantages, including assisting with calorie counting and ensuring that you have the right ingredients on hand for cooking recipes, quick meals, and snacks.

The following lists offer tips for incorporating the finest nutrient sources into your diet. You'll note that certain meals appear on multiple lists. An egg, for example, is heavy in fat but contains a significant quantity of protein. Nutrition calculators like MyFitnessPal and Cronometer can tell you how much of each nutrient a food has.

1. Healthy Fats

You don't notice a blood sugar or insulin surge when you eat primarily fat meals. As a result, try to get at least half of your daily calories from healthy fats such as the ones indicated.

- Fatty fish
- Nuts and seeds
- Avocados
- Eggs
- High-quality meats
- Cold-pressed oils (coconut oil, avocado oil, olive oil)

2. Healthy Proteins

The average person's protein requirements are met by modest protein consumption (15 to 25% of daily calories). Both plants and animal products can be used to make healthy choices.

Animal proteins

- Dairy products (cheese, milk, yogurt)
- Eggs
- Fish and seafood
- Meat (including organs) from beef, poultry, lamb, pork, and game animals

Plant proteins

- Beans and other legumes
- Whole grains
- Nuts and seeds

3. Healthy Carbohydrates

Even though all plant foods include carbs, they can nevertheless be included in a low-carb diet. You must choose intelligently to acquire the essential nutrients from plant foods without consuming too many carbohydrates. Lists of low-carb plant options can be found here.

Fruits

Fruits are high in nutrients, but if you have a slow metabolism, the natural sugars in fruits may make losing weight difficult. Limit the fruit intake and pick fruits with the lowest total carbohydrates if you have problems losing weight. Fruits are ranked based on the lowest and the highest net carbohydrates (net carbs are calculated based on a 3.5oz/100g meal).

Blackberries 4.3g	Oranges 9.4g
Coconuts 6.2g	Mandarins 11.5g
Raspberries 5.4g	Plums 10g
Strawberries 5.7g	Apples 11.4g
Avocados 1.8g	Pineapple 11.7g
Lemons 6.5g	Pears 12g
Cantaloupe 7.3g	Kiwi fruits 11.7g
Watermelon 7.2g	Blueberries 12.1g
Limes 7.7g	Mangoes 13.4g
Peaches 8g	Grapes 17.2g
Grapefruit 9.1g	Cherries 13.9g
Honeydew 8.3g	Bananas 20.2g
Apricots 9.1g	

Vegetables

Vegetables aren't all made equal. Some contain starch, making them more carbohydrate-dense than their non-starchy equivalents. Here you are a list of famous non-starchy veggies that are suitable for a low-carb diet.

Broccoli	Green beans
Brussels sprouts	Mushrooms
Asparagus	Leafy greens
Cabbage	Onions
Celery	Peppers
Cauliflower	Tomatoes

Cucumbers	Sugar snap peas and snow peas
Eggplants	Zucchini/summer squash
Collard greens	

Eat two cups of veggies baked in the oven, steamed, or sautéed to add variety to your diet. They become a delightful and healthy diet element when adding oil, salt, and other spices and herbs.

Because starchy vegetables have a high carb content per serving, they should be consumed in modest amounts, mainly on a low-carb diet. Examples include potatoes, green peas, starchy squashes, parsnips, and maize.

Because carrots are in the center of the non-starchy and starchy food groups, it's advisable to restrict your daily intake.

Nuts and seeds

To avoid the dangerous oils used in the commercial roasting, stay with raw varieties or roast your nuts. A list of nuts and seeds that are allowed in a low-carb diet may be found here.

Almonds	Pecans
Chia seeds	Pine nuts
Brazil nuts	Pumpkin seeds
Flaxseeds	Walnuts
Hazelnuts (a.k.a. filberts)	Sesame seeds
Hempseeds	Sunflower seeds
Macadamia nuts	

The flavor of nuts is enhanced when you toast them at home. The best overall color comes from oven-toasted nuts since they brown uniformly, although a pan will suffice.

Cook in a small-sized pan (without any fat) on medium flame, frequently turning until brown for up to 1/2 cup. Toast all nuts onto a baking sheet to 350°F for around 5 to 10 minutes, or till golden brown, for amounts over 1/2 cup. Toasted nuts can be frozen for up to 3 months in sealed containers.

3.4 How To Best Measure Your Intermittent Fasting Success

1. The Problem With The Scales

Have you ever felt like taking courage and stepping on the scales, only to be disappointed when the display doesn't reflect your expectations? Let's face it: many of us associate our happiness with a single value on a small screen because that's how we learned it and because it provides us with timely information. We can do that at any time and place because it is straightforward.

It's far too simple! Although most of us have always used weighing as our primary means of measurement, it is ineffective on its own.

This is because body weight is a more complicated phenomenon that reflects the sum of many variables and the various components of your body, such as bones, muscles, organs, blood, fat, water, etc. All of this is represented in the figure you refer to as your body weight.

Given that your body is made up of roughly 60% water and is influenced by various factors (including salt/caffeine intake, carbohydrate intake, time of day, sport, stress, and female cycle), any variation has a significant impact. Your scales can't possibly capture all of this.

2. Why Weight (Alone) Is Insufficient

Nothing else seems to happen for weeks, at least not on scales. But it may be already in the body! In the interim, you may have gained muscle and reduced fat without realizing it because your body weight hasn't changed. This information also opens the door to new ways of measuring your achievement!

That doesn't imply you should toss your scales out the window the next time you get a chance. It's neither a wicked device nor a notorious liar. However, it barely tells half the story, if at all. Other factors that are at least as essential as weight are ignored. You can't tell the difference between the trees and the timber.

3. So, What's The Point Of Measuring?

As a result, your weight should only be one piece of information regarding your body. If health is a 20-piece puzzle, body weight is one of them. As a result, we should strive to finish this puzzle. And measuring other regions of the body in this way is a potential move. It also doesn't require special equipment; anyone can perform it with a tape measure.

Even though the scale is at a standstill or driving you insane, measuring helps you see and capture the improvements. You could see how quickly you lose weight and, more importantly, where you lose it. This is something that nobody's fat analysis can perform because it can't tell the difference between "good" fat (neath the skin) and "bad" fat (on the belly). Measuring alone won't tell you anything about your body's composition, but it's a complicated issue. However, if your measures shrink while you retain the same weight, you've grown muscle while shedding fat. You'll start measuring your success in inches rather than pounds.

4. How Do I Know If I'm Measuring Correctly?

The ideal method is to take measurements of the bodily parts whose alterations you want to track. The chest, waist, and hips are more or less conventional, with the upper arms and thighs as a helpful addition. As with the scales, the same rule applies here: The quality of the work matters, not the quantity! Only measure yourself once or twice a month, ideally under the same conditions each time: In the morning or between meals, not immediately after that, and naked or in the same, form-fitting clothing.

Also, as ridiculous as it may sound, write down the results! It is the only way to see how far you've come. Then all you'll need is a soft and flexible fabric measuring tape.

And you're all set to go! Stand calmly in a mirror, close your legs, and breathe normally. It's much better if you can enlist the support of a friend, partner, or family member. It's best to start at the top and work your way down. Only measure one side of the body at a time, and don't overtighten or over-loosen the tape measure.

5. Where Should You Take Your Measurements?

The upper arm: measure the upper arm halfway between the elbow and shoulder joint at the broadest point.

Chest: at the broadest part of the chest, take a measurement. Most women have it at their nipple line.

Waist: one inch above the navel, measure your waist at its thinnest point. Close your legs, exhale slowly, and measure at the end of your exhalation.

Hip: close the legs, then measure the hip at the broadest point, at the level of the pelvic bones.

Thigh: at the widest part, midway between the knee and the hip, measure the thigh.

6. What Really Counts In Success Measuring

Are my measurements regular? YES, WITHOUT A DOUBT! Every human has a different body shape, just as the BMI (Body Mass Index) isn't very useful because it doesn't consider factors such as muscle mass or body composition and is only sometimes an accurate measure of health. BMI needs to adequately account for human diversity. A comparison with others is neither possible nor necessary!

Most likely, you're aiming for a specific weight or a set of supposedly perfect measurements. You don't need to get it out of the head for good. But consider this: Is it just the number that matters in the end? A few figures that will make you happy forever? Doubtful! Instead, it's about consciously perceiving physical changes and personally experiencing progress.

Success isn't measured in kilograms or inches. When you're proud of yourself and your progress and at ease in your skin, you've succeeded!

Chapter 4: Intermittent Fasting: Challenges and Solutions

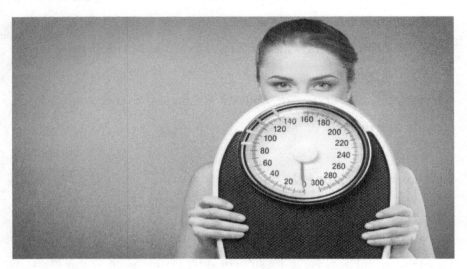

You are prepared to try Intermittent Fasting, but you should be aware of specific less-than-pleasant side effects you'll most likely encounter initially.

A qualified nutritionist, Stephanie Ferrari, stated: "Consider this: women do not go from couch potatoes to triathletes overnight. Any drastic changes in your environment require time for your body to adjust. When you stop eating for an extended time, you will experience various adverse effects." These can be excruciating at first, but if you learn how to deal with them, you can persist with Intermittent Fasting and reap the rewards.

4.1 Hunger Pains

When you eat five to six times daily, your body learns to anticipate food at specific times because of ghrelin. Stephanie remarked, "Ghrelin is the hormone that causes us to feel hungry. It is partially regulated by food consumption and usually peaks at breakfast, lunch, and dinner. Ghrelin levels may continue to rise when you initially begin fasting, and you will feel hungry".

It will take a lot of willpower at first. Days three to five are the most difficult, but you will eventually reach the start of your eating periods or not even feel hungry!

Dr. Luiza Petre, a nutrition and weight-loss expert and board-certified cardiologist, recommends drinking much water in the first week or two to keep your stomach full. This makes you feel more alert and help you break the habit of eating anything. Pound at least two glasses around 30 minutes after waking up. Drink additional two glasses or even more if you start to feel hungry. Intermittent Fasting teaches you that what you believed was hunger was most likely thirst or boredom.

Black tea and coffee can also help you feel full but may give you an acid stomach. Better to choose green tea, herbal teas, and infusions such as mallow, hibiscus, and chamomile. Get enough rest, stay busy, and avoid strenuous activities in the first few weeks, which can boost hunger. Preventing hunger also requires eating sufficiently the day before and getting your share of carbs, good fats, and protein.

4.2 Digestive Issues

If you undertake Intermittent Fasting, you might face digestive disorders, including constipation, nausea, diarrhea, and bloating.

The reduced food intake associated with various Intermittent Fasting regimens can have a significant impact on digestion, potentially leading to issues such as constipation and other undesirable side effects. In addition, dietary modifications related to Intermittent Fasting may result in bloating and diarrhea.

Because your stomach generates acid to aid digestion, you may suffer heartburn when you aren't eating (this side effect is not as prevalent as the others). This might range from slight discomfort to all-day burping to outright pain. This side effect should go away with time, so drink plenty of water, sleep on your side, and spicy foods, and avoid greasy, which could aggravate your heartburn. Consult your doctor if the problem persists.

Dehydration can exacerbate constipation, another typical side effect of Intermittent Fasting. As a result, it's critical to stay adequately hydrated when fasting intermittently. You can also avoid constipation by consuming nutrient-dense and fiber-rich foods.

4.3 Cravings

Intermittent Fasting triggers a physiological mechanism by which cravings decrease. The body's satiety hormone, leptin, primarily controls your appetite, which works by a negative feedback loop.

With the increase in leptin level, the appetite decreases.

Intermittent Fasting powers this negative feedback loop. When you fast, your leptin levels grow, and your hunger hormone lowers.

Your taste receptors will start to crave less and less super sweet food as your body secretes more and more leptin.

Intermittent Fasting is indeed a tool we can use to fight sugar cravings.

The matter may be different on a psychological level, as cravings are not always related to physiological needs.

To overcome cravings, do everything you can to avoid thinking about food. Drink a lot of water and keep yourself busy: your hormones will do the rest after a few days!

4.4 Headaches

Intermittent Fasting is sometimes associated with headaches. They usually happen in the first few days of the fasting regimen.

In a review published in 2020, researchers looked at 18 papers involving persons who practiced Intermittent Fasting. Some participants in the four studies who reported adverse effects indicated they had minor headaches.

Researchers have found that "fasting headaches" are mainly located in the frontal regions of our brain, with mild to somewhat moderate pain.

Furthermore, persons who suffer from headaches frequently are more prone to headaches when fasting than those who don't.

According to research, low blood sugar and caffeine withdrawal may lead to headaches while Intermittent Fasting.

Dull headaches, which come and go, are typical as your body adjusts to this new eating plan. Dehydration is a concern, so drink plenty of water during Fasting and feeding.

Low blood sugar levels could also trigger headaches and stress hormones the brain produces during Fasting. Your body will adjust to the new eating schedule over time, but try to stay as stress-free as possible.

4.5 Weakness

Expect to feel a little lazy in the first couple of days because your body no longer receives the consistent stream of fuel it used to get from consuming every day. To expend the least energy, keep your day as relaxing as possible. You should take a break from your workouts and perform gentle exercises like walking or yoga. Getting more sleep is also beneficial. According to studies, some people who practice multiple forms of Intermittent Fasting report weariness and low energy levels.

Intermittent Fasting can make you feel tired and weak due to low blood sugar. In addition, Intermittent Fasting may produce sleep disruptions in certain persons, resulting in fatigue throughout the day. But this is just a temporary situation: many studies have proven Intermittent Fasting reduces fatigue, especially when the body adapts to regular fasting intervals.

4.6 Sleep Disturbances

Intermittent Fasting may improve sleep quality by reinforcing circadian rhythms, which manage biological functions, including the sleep-wake cycle.

People who practice Intermittent Fasting may experience elevated levels of human growth hormone. This can lead to feeling more refreshed and restored after sleeping.

Even if Intermittent Fasting can enhance sleep quality, eating irregularly and late at night can disrupt sleep. Heavy meals before bedtime can upset the stomach, making it hard to fall asleep and affecting how rested you feel upon waking up.

Scheduling meals at least three hours before bedtime is an excellent strategy to avoid digestion disrupting sleep. On the other hand, you should stay hydrated to reduce hunger cravings and promote good sleep. Lastly, avoid caffeine and alcohol, which can disrupt sleep and negatively impact health. Choose healthy, nutrient-rich foods, and find a fasting schedule that works for you.

4.7 Dehydration

During the initial days of Fasting, the body expels a significant amount of water and salt through urine. This process, referred to as natural diuresis or fasting natriuresis, is responsible for this phenomenon.

If this occurs, you might become dehydrated and not restore the water and electrolytes lost through urine.

In addition, those who practice Intermittent Fasting might need to remember to drink or drink insufficiently. This is especially true when you initially start an Intermittent Fasting program.

Drink water during the day and check on the color of your urine to stay properly hydrated. It should ideally be the hue of pale lemonade. You may be dehydrated if your urine is black.

Fasting regularly may not be for everyone. Intermittent Fasting is not recommended for diabetes patients, pregnant, or even nursing mothers. Before beginning any diet plan or eating regimen, women with chronic conditions should always see their doctor. Finally, anyone with an eating disorder or at risk of developing one should avoid fasting.

These adverse effects should be noticed at all times. If you get dizzy from low blood sugar, if Fasting interferes with your ability to keep up with your duties, or if you develop an excessive preoccupation with eating, Intermittent Fasting might not be for you." You may have to break your fast and eat sooner than intended, or you may have to quit fasting entirely. It's a good idea to visit your doctor if you have any worries or troubles.

Chapter 5: 10 False Myths About Intermittent Fasting

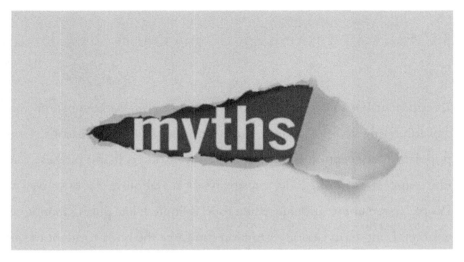

Intermittent Fasting recently gained considerable media attention. Some women, however, remain suspicious about whether it is beneficial, effective, or even healthful. Whether you're thinking about Intermittent Fasting or already doing it, it's critical to understand all the facts. If you do have the evidence, you will be able to fast appropriately. And if you fast appropriately, you'll have a better chance of experiencing weight loss, consistent energy, and reduced hunger sensations that have made Intermittent Fasting so famous.

There are several misunderstandings out there. Fasting myths, on the other side, are not based on reality. Instead, they are based on rumors, guesswork, and faith in ancient wisdom.

Let's debunk some of the most popular myths about Intermittent Fasting so you can make more informed decisions about using it as a health improvement technique.

5.1 Myth No 1: Intermittent Fasting Causes Starvation In The Body

Intermittent Fasting isn't starvation; it's a conscious food consumption gap for relatively brief periods for health and well-being reasons. One popular misconception about Intermittent Fasting is that it pushes your body into starvation mode, causing your metabolism to slow down. People starve unintentionally when food is limited, like during famine or conflict. Long-term calorie restriction can force the body to adapt to the lack of food and enter starvation mode, which indicates the body's metabolic rate is drastically reduced as a survival strategy. Intermittent Fasting is different from going hungry.

Intermittent Fasting avoids starvation mode adaption by alternating between consumption and restriction regularly. Fasting for a shorter time while alternating between Fasting and feasting enhances metabolic rate. Fasting for up to around 48 hours has been shown in studies to increase metabolism by 4 to 14%. Nevertheless, if you fast for an extended period, the results can reverse, lowering your metabolism.

5.2 Myth No 2: Intermittent Fasting Causes Muscle Loss

Malnutrition can cause muscle mass tissue to be lost. As a result, it appears reasonable to assume that skipping breakfast will cause muscle loss. On the other hand, Fasting has been shown to help preserve muscle mass compared to typical portion control. It has been suggested that a person must fast for five days or more in a row until a large amount of muscle can be used as fuel. Fasting may help this phase by boosting autophagy or eliminating old proteins in favor of newer ones, making them less likely to be weakened. Fasting combined with strength training has been found in studies to increase efficiency and muscular growth in trained muscles. Fasting causes a rise in growth hormones, which could explain some of this.

Just because you aren't eating regularly, especially protein, doesn't imply your body is going into "catabolic" mode, as many women believe. According to the hypothesis that the body requires a steady flow of proteins to heal, sustain, and generate muscle tissue, Fasting breaks down muscle fibers for energy.

Furthermore, a substantial amount of protein from the final meal before a 16-20 hour fast will almost certainly make proteins by the time you break the fast. Intermittent fasters frequently consume a substantial meal with 70+ grams of slow-absorbing protein before restarting their fast. Remember that prolonged Fasting can lead to muscle failure because "de novo gluconeogenesis" starts kicking in when muscle glycogen and amino acids are depleted. However, none of these scenarios will likely occur in 16-20 hours for women who fast intermittently and eat a large, nutritious meal before fasting again.

5.3 Myth No 3: Breakfast Deprivation Causes Weight Gain

Breakfast is frequently wrongly considered the most important meal of the day. Its deprivation is supposed to cause an increase in appetite, hunger symptoms, and weight gain. In a 16-week study of 283 obese or overweight persons, no weight difference existed between people who ate breakfast and those who didn't. Consequently, while there may be some individual differences, breakfast has no discernible effect on weight. Breakfast benefits many women, but this is optional for optimum health. According to controlled trials, there is minimal difference in weight loss between women who consume it and those who do not.

5.4 Myth No 4: Overeating Is A Result Of Fasting

After a fasting period, you'll be hungry. Many women feel that this hunger will cause them to binge. The evidence, on the other hand, disproves this concern. Most fasting trials enable participants to eat as much as they like, a process called ad-libitum eating. They can eat everything they want and yet lose weight. Many Intermittent Fasting approaches cause you to ingest fewer calories rather than more. Thanks to the reasonable calorie limit, you'll gradually lose weight without slowing your metabolic processes.

In multiple trials, Intermittent Fasting is a highly effective weight loss approach. Furthermore, no evidence skipping breakfast leads to weight gain. It's not to say you won't gain weight if you binge and overeat during your snacking sessions - you will. Intermittent Fasting is an efficient approach for weight reduction because it causes physiological changes in the body, such as a drop in insulin levels while raising metabolic rate, norepinephrine levels, and growth hormone concentrations.

The main conclusion is that you lose weight by creating a calorie imbalance over time, consuming less energy and spending more. (If you do the math backward, you'll have more weight.)

5.5 Myth No 5: Fasting For Short Periods Lowers The Metabolism But Eating Frequently Speeds It Up

Taking smaller and more frequent meals does not significantly increase your metabolism or help with weight loss. Indeed, the overall quantity of calories you take is more important than the number of meals you consume.

Without a doubt, your body expends calories digesting small, frequent meals – the scientific word for this is the thermic action of food (TEF). On average, the TEF consumes about 10% of your calorie intake, providing a minor metabolic boost.

According to new research, Intermittent Fasting speeds up your metabolism by lowering insulin levels and increasing blood levels of the human growth hormone and norepinephrine for short periods. These modifications may make it easier for you to burn fat and lose weight. Fasting each day for around 22 days did not decrease metabolic rate, but it did result in a 4% drop in fat mass, according to one study.

5.6 Myth No 6: It Is Best For Your Health To Eat Three Meals Per Day

Some women feel that eating three meals daily plus snacks is best for their health and weight loss, but this is untrue. Fasting, on the other hand, provides numerous health benefits. The three-meal-a-day plus-snacks diet does not cause the physiological changes in the body that have been shown to enhance the miraculous autophagy mechanism (the process of cellular repair).

Fasting for a short time triggers autophagy, which causes your cells to recycle old and defective proteins. Autophagy may aid in preventing aging, cancer, and neurological diseases such as Parkinson's and Alzheimer's. Indeed, several researchers suggest that frequent snacking or eating harms your health and increases your risk of illness. As a result, Intermittent Fasting is very far from unhealthy and has many advantages over regular eating patterns.

5.7 Myth No 7: To Grow Muscle, You Must Consume Protein Every Three Hours

More frequent protein consumption has been shown in studies not to affect muscle mass. It's a myth that you must eat protein every few hours and consume 20 to 30 grams of protein with any meal or snack to grow muscle. Intermittent Fasting can help women increase muscles and decrease weight. You should eat enough total proteins before and after the strength-training activities to grow muscles.

Gaining muscle requires a weight-training regimen for muscle acquisition while fasting and consuming sufficient calories to sustain muscle growth. Your body easily absorbs more than 30 grams of protein with every meal. Protein does not have to be consumed every 2 to 3 hours.

5.8 Myth No 8: The Brain Is Harmed By Intermittent Fasting

Blood sugar (also called glucose) is the brain's primary fuel, and it thrives on it. However, eating carbs once every hour is unnecessary for brain health: non-carbohydrate sources of glucose are easily converted into glucose by your body.

The brain uses ketones as an alternative energy source during Fasting, eliminating the need to provide the mind with a continual supply of dietary glucose.

You'll not only keep your mind working throughout those periods of Fasting if you force your body to burn fat stores and run on ketones sporadically, but you'll also boost cognition, strengthen neuron connections, and stave off dementia.

5.9 Myth No 9: Intermittent Fasting Results In Hazardous Blood Sugar Reductions

Intermittent Fasting helps prevent and reverse type 2 diabetes by stabilizing blood sugar levels. Your body is both a glucose storage and production machine. With strategic Intermittent Fasting, glucose levels usually stabilize, and the body undergoes significant changes and even reverses insulin-resistant disorders, such as diabetes, over time.

Hypoglycemia (extremely low blood glucose) is only used as a precaution in patients who have already been diagnosed with diabetes and diabetics who are receiving insulin or oral glucose-lowering medications. In these cases, you must obtain authorization from your healthcare provider to follow an intermittent fast.

5.10 Myth No 10: Intermittent Fasting On A Regular Basis Is Too Difficult

Fasting regularly might be challenging. Nonetheless, most individuals agree it is far more convenient than traditional diets. It doesn't require tiresome calorie counting (you either eat or don't), making the weight loss technique much easier for many women.

Furthermore, unlike traditional dieting, your sacrifice reaps many benefits, including improved weight and health and fat loss. Moreover, you are not bound by food limitations during your eating windows. When you eat less often, you spend less time and effort thinking about food shopping and preparing food. As a result, you can dedicate more time to your favorite activities.

Chapter 6: Healthy and Easy Recipes

Fasting between meals is a healthy approach to increasing energy, improving mental clarity, and losing weight. While not eating is one of its essential elements, what you consume in between is equally crucial. Here are some healthy breakfasts, main courses, snacks, and smoothie recipes you can enjoy while doing Intermittent Fasting.

BREAKFAST RECIPES

Oat-Egg Power Breakfast

Preparation Time: 15 minutes

Servings: 1

Nutrition Facts: Calories 191; Total Fat 5g; Carbohydrates 30g; Protein 7g

Ingredients:

o   1 egg

o   1 cup of oat milk

o   2 dates

o   ½ cup of oats

o   1 tablespoon of oat flour

o   1 tablespoon of almonds

o   1 tablespoon of fresh blueberries

o   A pinch of Himalayan salt

Instructions:

⇒   In a mixer, combine oat milk and dates.

⇒   Now, place the mixture inside a pot with 1 egg and bring to a boil.

⇒   Start mixing it after a while and add the oat flour and oats.

⇒   Combine the ingredients, spread the blueberries and almonds on top, and season with salt.

Scrambled Egg Breakfast

Preparation Time: 10 minutes

Servings: 1

Nutrition Facts: Calories 161; Total Fat 7.5g; Carbohydrates 14g; Protein 10g

Ingredients:

o   1 medium Egg

o   1 ounce of low-fat cheddar cheese

o   1 ounce of avocado

o   ½ cup of egg whites

o   ½ cup of white mushrooms, sliced

o   3-5 fresh mint leaves

Instructions:

⇒ Combine egg yolk and egg whites in a mixing bowl. Spray a skillet with cooking spray and cook till the eggs are no longer runny.

⇒ Sauté the mushrooms in a separate skillet with butter-flavored cooking spray.

⇒ Avocado should be sliced, and cheese should be shredded.

⇒ Melt the cheese on top of the eggs. Add cooked mushrooms and sliced avocado.

⇒ Decorate with mint leaves and serve.

Chia Seed Banana Blueberry Delight

Preparation Time: 25 minutes

Servings: 2

Nutrition Facts: Calories 141; Total Fat 6g; Carbohydrates 20g; Protein 2g

Ingredients:

o   1 cup of yogurt

o   1 banana

o   ½ cup of blueberries

o   ½ cup of raspberries

o   ¼ cup of chia seeds

o   1 teaspoon of vanilla extract

o   ½ teaspoon of cinnamon

o   A pinch of salt

Instructions:

⇒ Remove the skin off the banana and cut it into rings of medium thickness. You can either mash them up or leave the lumps alone if you prefer it that way.

⇒ Wash the blueberries thoroughly with water.

⇒ Soak the chia seeds in water for a period of 30 minutes.

⇒ Drain the chia seeds and place them in a mixing dish.

⇒ Combine with yogurt, salt, cinnamon, and vanilla and whisk well.

⇒ Add the blueberries, banana and raspberries just before serving.

Breakfast Spinach Frittata

Preparation Time: 15 minutes

Servings: 2

Nutrition Facts: Calories 325; Total Fat 23g; Carbohydrates 9g; Protein 20g

Ingredients:

o   2 eggs

o   1 ounce of spinach

o   Salt and black pepper to taste

o   1 tablespoon of olive oil extra virgin

o   2 ounces of low fat mozzarella, shredded

o   Hot sauce (optional)

Instructions:

⇒   Cook the spinach using olive oil in a small-sized nonstick frying pan over a medium flame until wilted.

⇒   In a bowl, whisk the eggs and pour them into the pan. Season with salt and pepper, then top with mozzarella.

⇒   Cook for around 4 minutes or till bottom is lightly browned, then flip and cook for another 4 minutes or until bottom is lightly browned (around another 3-4 minutes).

⇒   Drizzle with hot sauce or garnish as desired after transferring to a platter. Serve right away and enjoy!

Blueberry and Oat Pancakes with Cinnamon

Preparation Time: 20 minutes

Servings: 2

Nutrition Facts: Calories 253; Total Fat 12g; Carbohydrates 29g; Protein 7g

Ingredients:

o   1 ounce of porridge oats

o   1 large free-range egg

o   3 ounces of fresh or frozen blueberries

o   1 tablespoon of self-rising flour

o   ½ cup of skimmed milk

o   1 ½ teaspoons of Splenda

o   ½ teaspoon of ground cinnamon

o   low fat cooking spray

Instructions:

⇒   Stir the egg white in a clean bowl till it is stiff and holds peaks. In a separate bowl, whisk together the egg yolk, sweetener, flour, oats, cinnamon, and milk.

⇒ With a metal spoon, gently stir the egg whites into the oat and flour mixture, taking care to retain as many of the light egg white content as possible.

⇒ Spray a nonstick frying pan with low-fat oil, around 2 to 3 sprays, and heat. To form tiny pancakes, spoon tablespoons of pancake batter into the frying pan and cook for 2-3 minutes, until puffed up, before carefully turning over and cooking on the other side till golden. (You should be able to make around 7 to 8 pancakes from the batter.)

⇒ Set the pancakes on a platter and cover with a tea towel to keep it warm while you finish the rest.

⇒ Meanwhile, in a small saucepan, slowly cook the blueberries with approximately a tablespoon of water and the sweetener, stirring constantly until the fruit is mushy and broken down.

⇒ Serve the hot blueberry sauce with the pancakes and a sprinkling of more cinnamon, if desired.

Delicious Stuffed Peppers

Preparation Time: 45 minutes

Servings: 2

Nutrition Facts: Calories 306; Total Fat 23g; Carbohydrates 10g; Protein 16g

Ingredients:

o   1 large tomato, diced
o   1 bell pepper sliced in half
o   6 ounces of ground turkey
o   1 slice of bacon, cut into ½" strips
o   1 tablespoon of onion, chopped
o   1 teaspoon chili powder
o   ½ teaspoon of ground cumin
o   ½ teaspoon of dried oregano
o   ½ teaspoon of paprika
o   salt and ground black pepper to taste
o   ½ cup of chicken broth

- o   2 tablespoons of shredded cheddar
- o   1 tablespoon of green onion, thinly sliced

Instructions:

⇒ Preheat oven to 350°.

⇒ Add bacon to a non-stick skillet over medium heat and cook for 5 minutes. Place on a paper towel-lined dish and put aside.

⇒ Add onion to the same skillet and brown them for about 5 minutes. Add turkey and cook for 5 minutes, frequently stirring with a wooden spoon.

⇒ Spread the spices and season with salt and pepper.

⇒ Stir in broth and tomatoes and bring to a simmer. Cook for another 15 minutes.

⇒ Place the bell pepper halves in a large baking dish and fill them with the ground turkey mixture. Top with bacon and cheddar, then bake for 15 minutes. Remove from the oven and let cool for 5 minutes. Garnish with green onions and serve.

High Protein Breakfast Cups

Preparation Time: 25 minutes

Servings: 4

Nutrition Facts: Calories 361; Total Fat 26g; Carbohydrates 1g; Protein 27g

Ingredients:

- o   15 ounces ground beef
- o   ½ teaspoon fresh thyme
- o   1 garlic clove, minced
- o   1/8 teaspoon paprika
- o   1/8 teaspoon ground cumin
- o   a pinch of kosher salt and ground black pepper
- o   1 cup of fresh spinach, chopped
- o   ½ cup low-fat cheddar cheese, shredded
- o   4 eggs
- o   1 teaspoon chives, chopped

Instructions:

⇒ Preheat oven to 400°F.

⇒ Add ground beef, garlic, thyme, paprika, cumin, salt, and pepper in a medium-sized mixing bowl. Mix well until combined.

⇒ Add a small amount of ground beef mixture to each muffin tin, then create a cup by pressing the sides.

⇒ Divide spinach and cheese between the cups. Crack an egg over each cup and season with salt and pepper.

⇒ Bake for about 20 minutes, until eggs are set, and sausage is cooked through.

⇒ Garnish with chives, then serve.

Berry Nutty Yogurt Bowl

Preparation Time: 3 minutes

Servings: 1

Nutrition Facts: Calories 194; Total Fat 5g; Carbohydrates 13g; Protein 23g

Ingredients:

o   1 cup fat-free Greek yogurt,
o   1/2 cup mixed berries
o   1 tbsp chopped almonds

Instructions:

⇒ Top Greek yogurt with mixed berries and chopped almonds.

⇒ Serve immediately and enjoy!

Green Toast

Preparation Time: 10 minutes

Servings: 2

Nutrition Facts: Calories 226; Total Fat 14g; Carbohydrates 17g; Protein 10g

Ingredients:

o   2 slices whole grain bread
o   1 avocado
o   2 eggs

Instructions:

⇒ Toast bread and mash avocado on top.

⇒ Poach egg and place on top of avocado toast.

⇒ Serve warm.

Berry Oatmeal Delight

Preparation Time: 10 minutes

Servings: 2

Nutrition Facts: Calories 168; Total Fat 5g; Carbohydrates 23g; Protein 5g

Ingredients:

o   1/2 cup rolled oats
o   2 cups unsweetened almond milk
o   1 cup mixed berries

Instructions:

⇒ Cook oats according to package instructions with almond milk..

⇒ Top with mixed berries

⇒ Serve warm.

Spinach Mushroom Scramble

Preparation Time: 15 minutes

Servings: 2

Nutrition Facts: Calories 166; Total Fat 11g; Carbohydrates 4g; Protein 13g

Ingredients:

o   4 eggs
o   4 cups spinach leaves
o   1/2 cup mushrooms
o   1 tsp olive oil

Instructions:

⇒ Whisk eggs in a bowl.

⇒ Sauté spinach and mushrooms in a oiled skillet until wilted.

⇒ Add eggs to skillet and scramble until cooked through.

⇒ Serve hot or warm.

Overnight Chia Pudding

Preparation Time: 10 minutes plus overnight chilling

Servings: 2

Nutrition Facts: Calories 200; Total Fat 11g; Carbohydrates 22g; Protein 5g

Ingredients:

o 1/4 cup chia seeds

o 1 cup unsweetened almond milk (or any milk of your choice)

o 1 tablespoon honey or maple syrup

o 1/2 teaspoon vanilla extract

o 1/4 cup mixed berries for topping

o 1 tbsp shredded coconut

Instructions:

⇒ In a bowl, combine chia seeds, almond milk, honey or maple syrup, and vanilla extract. Stir well to combine.

⇒ Let the mixture sit for 5 minutes, then give it another stir to break up any clumps of chia seeds.

⇒ Cover the bowl and refrigerate overnight or for at least 3 hours, allowing the chia seeds to absorb the liquid and thicken.

⇒ When ready to serve, give the chia pudding a good stir to redistribute the seeds.

⇒ Divide the chia pudding into two serving bowls or glasses.

⇒ Top with mixed berries and shredded coconut before enjoying.

MAIN COURSE RECIPES

Tempting Fish Soup

Preparation Time: 35 minutes

Servings: 4

Nutrition Facts: Calories 256; Total Fat 4; Carbohydrates 10g; Protein 38g

Ingredients:

o   1 cup of chicken broth

o   ½ onion, chopped

o   ¼ cup of black olives, sliced

o   ½ cup of dry white wine

o   ½ green bell pepper, chopped

o   1 teaspoon of dried basil

o   2 cloves of garlic, minced

o   1 pound of medium shrimp, peeled and deveined

o   1 can of diced tomatoes (14.5 ounces)

o   ½ teaspoon of ground black pepper

o   2 1/2 ounces of canned mushrooms

o   2 bay leaves

o   1 pound of cod fillets, cubed

o   ½ cup of orange juice

o   ½ teaspoon of crushed fennel seed

o   2 tablespoons of fresh parsley

Instructions:

⇒ Toss the onion, green bell pepper, garlic, chicken broth, mushrooms, diced tomato, olives, orange juice, wine, bay leaves, fennel seeds, dried basil, and pepper together in a large non-stick frying pan or a wok. Cook the vegetables at medium heat for 20 minutes, or till they are soft.

⇒ Add the shrimp and cod to the pan. Cook over medium heat for around 10 minutes, or till the shrimp are completely opaque. Bay leaves should be taken out and thrown away.

⇒ Garnish with parsley and serve hot.

Loaded Barley Salad with Fresh Veggies

Preparation Time: 35 minutes

Servings: 4

Nutrition Facts: Calories 324; Total fat 13g; Carbohydrates 48g; Protein 8g

Ingredients:

o 1 cup of cucumber, diced

o 1/4 cup of feta cheese

o 1 cup of pearl barley

o 1/4 cup of red onion, diced

o 3 cups of water

o Fresh parsley for garnish

o 1/2 teaspoon of salt

o 1/3 cup of Kalamata olives

o 1 cup of halved grape tomatoes

o 1 diced bell pepper

o ½ cup of Greek salad dressing

Instructions:

⇒ A big saucepan of salted water should be brought to a boil. After adding the barley, reduce the flame to low and cover the pot with a lid. Cook the barley for a total of 15 minutes, till it is soft. Allow any surplus liquid to drain and cool completely.

⇒ Cut the vegetables and place them in a large mixing bowl while the barley cooks.

⇒ Add the chilled barley dressing to the mixing bowl. Toss everything together well.

⇒ Serve with parsley and feta cheese crumbles on top. Chill for around 1 hour before serving.

Tuna Salad

Preparation Time: 35 minutes

Servings: 1

Nutrition Facts: Calories 302; Total fat 11g; Carbohydrates 18g; Protein 33g

Ingredients:

o 3 tablespoons of low-fat mayonnaise

o 8 chopped olives

o Salt and ground black pepper, to taste

o 1 can of tuna in water (6 ounces), drained

o 2 tablespoons of hummus spread

o 1 teaspoon of dried oregano, to taste

o 1 cup of lettuce

o 1 tomato, sliced

Instructions:

⇒ With a fork, flake the tuna into a small-sized bowl. Combine the low-fat mayonnaise, olives, and hummus. To taste, season with salt, oregano, and pepper.

⇒ Combine all of the ingredients in a medium mixing bowl and chill for 30 minutes.

⇒ Put lettuce on a serving plate. Spread the tuna sauce and garnish with tomato slices before serving.

Chicken with Basil-Lemon Gravy

Preparation Time: 35 minutes

Servings: 2

Nutrition Facts: Calories 326; Total Fat 11g; Carbohydrates 6g; Protein 46g

Ingredients:

⇒ 1 tablespoon of all-purpose flour

⇒ 1/2 cup of chicken stock

⇒ 2 chicken breast halves, boned and skinned

⇒ 1 tablespoon of butter

⇒ 1 tablespoon of chopped fresh basil

⇒ 1 tablespoon of fresh lemon juice

⇒ ½ tablespoon of lemon zest

⇒ 1 tablespoon of fresh parsley

Instructions:

⇒ On a chopping board, arrange the chicken breasts. With the smooth side of a meat mallet, flatten gently. Make a fine flour coating on the chicken on all sides. In a large-sized skillet over a medium-high flame, melt the butter. In a skillet, cook chicken breasts until lightly browned on both sides, about 6 minutes per side. Remove the fillets from the pan and set aside.

⇒ Meanwhile, add the chicken stock, basil, fresh lemon juice, and lemon zest in the same pan. With the lid on, cook for about 5 minutes. After adding the cooked chicken, simmer for another 5 minutes.

⇒ Transfer the chicken to a serving tray and simmer for another 5 minutes, or until the sauce thickens. Pour the sauce over the chicken and toss to coat.

⇒ Sprinkle with fresh parsley and serve.

Tempting Chili Garlic Chicken

Preparation Time: 30 minutes+ 2 hours

Servings: 4

Nutrition Facts: Calories 265; Total Fat 18g; Carbohydrates 1g; Protein 24g

Ingredients:

o   4 breast fillets of chicken

o   2 tablespoons of olive oil extra-virgin

o   ¼ teaspoon of salt

o   1/2 teaspoon of onion powder

o   1 tablespoon of red chili flakes

o   1/4 teaspoon of ground black pepper

o   1 teaspoon of minced garlic

Instructions:

⇒ In a large mixing bowl, combine the garlic, olive oil, onion powder, chili flakes, salt, and pepper. Combine all of the ingredients thoroughly. After that, add the chicken fillets. The marinating process should take at least two hours.

⇒ Cook the fillets in the nonstick pan for about 15 minutes over medium heat, or till the marinated chicken fillets are completely cooked.

Greek-Style Feta Chicken

Preparation Time: 30 minutes+ 4 hours

Servings: 4

Nutrition Facts: Calories 315; Total Fat 20g; Carbohydrates 4g; Protein 31g

Ingredients:

o   1/2 cup of feta cheese, crumbled

o   4 halves chicken breast boneless and skinless

- o 1/4 cup of fresh parsley, chopped
- o 2 tablespoons of olive oil extra-virgin
- o 1 cup of plain Greek yogurt
- o 2 cloves of garlic, minced
- o ¼ teaspoon of ground black pepper
- o ½ teaspoon of dried oregano
- o 10 black olives, deseeded and halved

Instructions:

⇒ In a mixing dish, combine the minced garlic, Greek yogurt, oregano, and black pepper. The yogurt marinade should be applied to both sides of the chicken. Refrigerate in an airtight jar for 4 hours.

⇒ In a nonstick pan, preheat 2 tablespoons olive oil over medium heat. After taking the chicken from the yogurt marinade, place it on the pan.

⇒ Cook on one side for 6 minutes before turning and sprinkle with feta cheese. Cook for an additional 5 minutes, or until the chicken is no longer pink in the center and the juices flow clear.

⇒ Sprinkle with olives and serve.

Tempting Chicken Satay

Preparation Time: 30 minutes

Servings: 2

Nutrition Facts: Calories 486; Total Fat 26g; Carbohydrates 16g; Protein 51g

Ingredients:

- o 2 chicken breasts skinless and boneless, cut them lengthwise into strips

For the Marinade:

- o 2 tablespoons of soy sauce
- o 2 tablespoons of tomato sauce

o   1 tablespoon of peanut oil

o   1 cloves of garlic, minced

o   ¼ teaspoon of ground black pepper

o   ¼ teaspoon of ground cumin

For the Peanut Sauce:

o   1 tablespoon of onion finely chopped

o   1 teaspoon of sugar

o   1 tablespoon of peanut butter

o   1 clove of garlic, minced

o   ½ lemon, sliced

o   1 teaspoon of peanut oil

o   1 teaspoon of soy sauce

o   ¼ cup of water

Instructions:

⇒ Cover wooden skewers in water in a shallow bowl. Allow for soaking time of 20 minutes.

⇒ Arrange the chicken strips in a mixing bowl. In a small cup, combine the soy sauce, tomato sauce, peanut oil, garlic, cumin, and pepper. Toss the chicken strips in the sauce to evenly coat all sides.

⇒ Allow 15 minutes for the marinating process.

⇒ Make the peanut sauce in the meantime. 1 tablespoon oil heated over medium-high heat in a hot skillet Mix the onion and garlic.

⇒ Cook, stirring occasionally, for 4 minutes, or until onion is soft and translucent.

⇒ In a mixing bowl, combine the peanut butter, soy sauce, sweetener, and water. Make a thorough mix.

⇒ Cook for an additional 5 minutes, or until the sauce has thickened slightly. Remove the pan from the flame and squeeze the lemon juice into it.

⇒ Using a skewer, thread each chicken strip. On the grill, cook for about 20 minutes. Serve the satay skewers with the peanut sauce for dipping right away.

Shrimp Skewers with Cilantro Lime

Preparation Time: 30 minutes

Servings: 4

Nutrition Facts: Calories 150; Total Fat 8g; Carbohydrates 3g; Protein 16g

Ingredients:

o   3 garlic cloves, minced

o   1 jalapeno pepper ,seeded and minced

o   ¼ teaspoon of salt

o   1/3 cup of chopped fresh cilantro

o   2 tablespoons of olive oil extra-virgin

o   1 pound of shrimp (16-20 per pound) peeled, deveined, and uncooked

o   Lime slices

o   ¼ teaspoon of ground cumin

o   1/3 cup of lime juice

o   1 ½ teaspoons of grated lime zest

o   ¼ teaspoon of pepper

Instructions:

⇒ Combine cilantro, lime juice, grated lime zest, jalapeño pepper, extra-virgin olive oil, salt, minced garlic cloves, cumin, and pepper in a large-sized mixing bowl. Set aside for 15 minutes after tossing the shrimp in the mixture.

⇒ Thread the shrimp and lime slices onto skewers. Arrange the vegetables on the grill.

⇒ Cook for around 10 to 15 minutes on the grill. After the cooking half-time has passed, flip the kebabs.

Flavorsome Almond-Crusted Tilapia

Preparation Time: 30 minutes

Servings: 4

Nutrition Facts: Calories 404; Total Fat 20g; Carbohydrates 22g; Protein 34g

Ingredients:

o ½ cup of almond flour

o 1 cup of breadcrumbs

o 4 tilapia fish fillet

o ½ teaspoon of garlic powder

o ½ teaspoon of onion powder

o 2 tablespoons of olive oil

o 1 teaspoon of lemon pepper

o 2 whole eggs

o ¼ cup of parmesan cheese, grated

o ¼ teaspoon of Kosher salt

Instructions:

⇒ In a mixing dish, combine the lemon pepper, salt, and eggs; set aside.

⇒ Combine the almond flour, onion powder, parmesan, breadcrumbs, and garlic powder in a small container.

⇒ Coat each fillet in each mixture, then in the breadcrumb mixture, making sure both sides are properly coated.

⇒ Place them in a nonstick frying pan that has been preheated with olive oil.

⇒ Cook over medium heat for around 15 to 20 minutes, flipping once halfway through the cooking time.

ill Salmon Spiced Cumin

Preparation Time: 30 minutes

Servings: 4

Nutrition Facts: Calories 281; Total Fat 20g; Carbohydrates 2g; Protein 23g

Ingredients:

o   2 tablespoons of olive oil

o   1 teaspoon of ground cumin

o   2 tablespoons of lime juice

o   1 teaspoon of fresh dill weed, chopped

o   1 lb. of salmon belly

o   Salt and freshly ground black pepper

o   1 teaspoon of garlic powder

Instructions:

⇒ Combine lime juice, garlic powder, olive oil, and dill in a small-sized dish.

⇒ Warm a large nonstick skillet.

⇒ Place the salmon belly. Season with pepper and salt to taste after drizzling the olive oil mixture over both sides.

⇒ Cook for approximately 15 minutes, or till golden brown. Turn them over halfway through the cooking time.

Easy Beef Stew

Preparation Time: 1 hour and 20 minutes

Servings: 4

Nutrition Facts: Calories 317; Total Fat 22g; Carbohydrates 7g; Protein 23g

Ingredients:

- 1 pound of beef chuck roast, cut into 1" pieces
- A pinch of Kosher salt
- Freshly ground black pepper
- 1 tablespoon of olive oil
- 6 ounces of Portobello mushrooms, sliced
- 1 onion, chopped
- 1 carrot, peeled and cut into rounds
- 1 stalk of celery, sliced
- 1 garlic clove, minced
- 1 tablespoon of tomato paste
- 3 cups of low-sodium beef broth
- ½ tablespoon fresh thyme
- 1 teaspoon freshly chopped rosemary

Instructions:

⇒ Season the beef well with salt and pepper.

⇒ Heat oil in a large pot over a medium flame.

⇒ Add beef and sear on all sides until golden, about 3 minutes per side.

⇒ To the same pot, stir in mushrooms and cook until golden and crispy, for about 5 minutes. Add onion, carrots, and celery and cook for five more minutes.

⇒ Add garlic, tomato paste and cook for another minute.

⇒ Add broth, thyme, rosemary, and beef to the pot and bring to a boil. Reduce the flame and simmer until the meat is tender, from 45 to 55 minutes.

Beef & Cheese Lettuce Wraps

Preparation Time: 20 minutes

Servings: 4

Nutrition Facts: Calories 382; Total Fat 26g; Carbohydrates 4g; Protein 32g

Ingredients:

- 1 tablespoon olive oil
- 1 small white onion, thinly sliced

- 1 bell pepper, thinly sliced
- ½ teaspoon of oregano
- Kosher salt and ground black pepper
- 1 lb. skirt steak, thinly sliced
- 1 cup of provolone, shredded
- 4 large butterhead lettuce leaves
- 1 tablespoon of fresh parsley, chopped
- ½ tablespoon fresh thyme

Instructions:

⇒ Heat one tablespoon of oil in a large nonstick skillet over medium heat. Add onion and bell peppers and season with oregano, salt, and pepper. Cook, often stirring, for about 10 minutes. Remove peppers and onions from skillet and heat remaining oil in skillet.

⇒ Add steak and cook for 2-4 minutes on each side.

⇒ Put the onion mixture back into the skillet and toss to combine. Sprinkle provolone, then cover and cook until the cheese has melted, for about 1 minute. Remove from heat.

⇒ Arrange lettuce leaves on a serving dish. Spread the steak mixture over each piece of lettuce. Garnish with parsley and serve warm.

Pork Tenderloin with Leeks

Preparation Time: 40 minutes
Servings: 2
Nutrition Facts: Calories 180; Total Fat 18g; Carbohydrates 5g; Protein 13g

Ingredients:
- 1 tablespoon extra-virgin oil
- 1 leek, sliced
- 1 tablespoon mustard seeds
- 8-ounce Pork tenderloin
- 1 tablespoon cumin seeds
- 1 tablespoon dry mustard
- 1 tablespoon of butter

Instructions:
⇒ Preheat the oven to 375°F.
⇒ In a non-stick skillet, heat mustard and cumin seeds until they start to pop (3–5 minutes).
⇒ Grind seeds with a blender and then mix in the dry mustard.
⇒ Coat the pork on both sides with the mustard blend and add to a baking tray—Bake for 30 minutes or until cooked through. Turn once halfway through.
⇒ Remove and set aside.
⇒ Heat the butter in a pan over medium heat and cook the leeks for 5–6 minutes or until soft.
⇒ Serve warm the pork tenderloin on a bed of leeks.

Cheese-Stuffed Mushrooms

Preparation Time: 35 minutes
Servings: 2
Nutrition Facts: Calories 410; Total Fat 26g; Carbohydrates 12g; Protein 19g

Ingredients:
o   4 Portobello mushrooms
o   2 tablespoons extra-virgin olive oil
o   1 onion, chopped
o   1 garlic clove, minced
o   1 cup red cabbage, shredded
o   Sea Salt and ground black pepper
o   3 tablespoons water
o   ½ cup of cheddar cheese, shredded

Instructions:
⇒ Preheat the oven to 400°F.
⇒ Rinse the mushrooms briefly and pat dry. Remove the stems and discard. Set aside.
⇒ In a nonstick skillet, heat the olive oil over medium heat. Sautv© onion and garlic for 2 minutes, stirring.
⇒ Add cabbage salt and pepper for 3 minutes, stirring frequently.
⇒ Add water, cover, and steam the cabbage for 5 minutes.
⇒ Transfer the vegetables into a medium bowl; let cool for 10 minutes, then stir in the cheese.

⇒ Put the mushroom caps on a baking tray and divide the filling among the mushrooms-

⇒ Bake for 15 minutes, then serve hot or warm.

Cheesy Cauliflower Comfort

Preparation Time: 35 minutes

Servings: 4

Nutrition Facts: Calories 152; Total Fat 12g; Carbohydrates 5g; Protein 7g

Ingredients:

o   1 head cauliflower

o   1/2 cup reduced-fat cream

o   1/2 cup cheddar cheese, shredded

o   1/4 cup parmesan cheese, grated

o   Salt and pepper to taste

Instructions:

⇒ Preheat the oven to 375°F.

⇒ Cut the cauliflower into small florets and steam until tender.

⇒ In a large bowl, whisk together the reduced-fat cream, cheddar cheese, and parmesan cheese.

⇒ Add the steamed cauliflower to the bowl and stir until well coated.

⇒ Season with salt and pepper to taste.

⇒ Transfer the mixture to a baking dish and bake for 20-25 minutes or until golden brown.

Vegan Chili

Preparation Time: 40 minutes

Servings: 4

Nutrition Facts: Calories 286; Total Fat 9g; Carbohydrates 13g; Protein 39g

Ingredients:

o   1 tsp olive oil

o   1/2 onion, chopped

o   2 cloves garlic, minced

o   1 green bell pepper, chopped

o   1 jalapeño pepper, seeded and minced

- o 1 tbsp chili powder
- o Salt and pepper to taste
- o 1 cup vegetable broth
- o Half can diced tomatoes (7 oz)

Instructions:

⇒ Heat olive oil in a large pot over medium heat.

⇒ Add onion and garlic; cook until onion is translucent.

⇒ Add green bell pepper and jalapeño pepper; cook for 10 minutes or until peppers are tender.

⇒ Add chili powder; cook for one minute.

⇒ Add salt and pepper to taste.

⇒ Add vegetable broth, diced tomatoes, meat substitute and bring to a boil.

⇒ Reduce heat and simmer for about 20 minutes.

Zucchini Noodle Alfredo Delight

Preparation Time: 40 minutes

Servings: 4

Nutrition Facts: Calories 112; Total Fat 9g; Carbohydrates 3g; Protein 5g

Ingredients:

- o two medium-sized zucchinis, spiralized
- o 2 tbsp reduced-fat cream
- o 2 tbsp Parmesan cheese, grated
- o 1 garlic clove
- o 1 tbsp butter
- o Salt and pepper to taste
- o Parsley leaves – for garnishing
- o Salt and pepper to taste

Instructions:

⇒ In a pan melt butter over medium heat.

⇒ Add garlic and sauté for a minute.

⇒ Add reduced-fat cream and parmesan cheese to the pan.

⇒ Stir continuously until the cheese melts completely.

⇒ Add salt and black pepper.

⇒ Add zucchini noodles to the pan and toss them well with the sauce.

⇒ Cook for about two minutes or until the zucchini noodles are tender.

⇒ Garnish with parsley leaves.

Stuffed Zucchini Boats

Preparation Time: 30 minutes

Servings: 2

Nutrition Facts: Calories 192; Total fat 12g; Carbohydrates 12g; Protein 9g

Ingredients:

o   1/4 medium onion, chopped

o   1 tbsp of pine nuts

o   2 tbsp of feta cheese, crumbled

o   1 teaspoon of dried basil

o   3 medium-sized zucchini

o   2 tablespoons of diced green olives

o   1 teaspoon of dried oregano

o   2 chopped cloves of garlic

o   ½ cup of grated Asiago cheese, divided

Instructions:

⇒ Place an oven rack roughly 6 inches away from the heat source to preheat the oven's broiler.

⇒ Remove the zucchini ends and cut each squash in half lengthwise. Scrape the seeds out of the squash and place them in a mixing bowl.

⇒ Combine the onion, feta cheese, olives, basil, garlic, pine nuts, 1/2 cup Asiago cheese, and oregano in a large mixing bowl. Fill the zucchini shells with the mixture. Place the zucchini boats on a baking sheet and sprinkle with a little amount of Asiago cheese.

⇒ Cook under a hot broiler for around 10 minutes, or till the cheese has browned.

Spinach and Cheese Stuffed Mushrooms

Preparation Time: 30 minutes

Servings: 4

Nutrition Facts: Calories 195; Total fat 9g; Carbohydrates 20g; Protein 11g

Ingredients:

o 5 ounces frozen spinach chopped

o 1 onion chopped

o 2 tbsp of butter

o 1 package of mushrooms, stems removed (8 ounces)

o 2 tbsp of dry breadcrumbs

o 2 tbsp of Italian-style salad dressing

o 3 tbsp reduced-fat cream cheese

o 2 tbsp of Parmesan cheese, grated

o 1 garlic clove, minced

Instructions:

⇒ Apply Italian dressing on all sides of each mushroom cap.

⇒ Cook for around 5 minutes at 390°F or till mushrooms are tender. Remove the mushrooms from the oven but leave the oven door ajar.

⇒ Melt butter in a skillet on medium-high flame and cook garlic and onion for around 6 to 8 minutes, or till onion softens. Combine the parmesan cheese, spinach, cream cheese, and 3 tablespoons of bread crumbs.

⇒ Before topping with the leftover bread crumbs, evenly spread the spinach mixture among the mushroom caps. Return the mushrooms to the oven for a final 10 minutes of cooking, or till golden brown on top.

SNACK RECIPES

Almond-Garlic Crackers

Preparation Time: 30 minutes

Servings: 4

Nutrition Facts: Calories 72; Total fat 5.7g; Carbohydrates 3.1g; Protein 3.1g

Ingredients:

- ½ cup of the almond meal
- ¼ teaspoon of salt
- 1 teaspoon of garlic powder
- 3 tablespoons of Parmesan cheese, grated
- ½ cup of water
- ½ cup of ground flax seed

Instructions:

⇒ Preheat the oven at 400°F.

⇒ In a medium-sized mixing bowl, combine ground flaxseed, almond meal, water, grated Parmesan cheese, garlic powder, and salt. Allow 3–5 minutes for the water to settle and the dough to firm up.

⇒ Cover the dough with waxed paper or plastic wrap and place it on the prepared baking sheet. With a rolling pin or your fingertips, flatten the dough to 1/8-inch thickness. Leaving waxed paper out of the equation.

⇒ Using a knife, make indentations in the dough to demonstrate where the crackers will be torn apart.

⇒ Bake for around 15 minutes, or till gently brown.

Pizza Muffins

Preparation Time: 30 minutes

Servings: 4

Nutrition Facts: Calories 117; Total Fat 8g; Carbohydrates 4g; Protein 8g

Ingredients:

o   2 medium zucchini, grated
o   1 tablespoon of butter, melted
o   2 large whole eggs
o   1 cup of mozzarella, grated
o   ¼ teaspoon of salt
o   2 tablespoons of coconut flour
o   ½ teaspoon of black pepper

For the topping:

o   1 oz. slices of pepperoni
o   2/3 cup of mozzarella, grated
o   1/4 cup of marinara sauce
o   1 teaspoon of the Italian seasoning

Instructions:

⇒ Preheat the oven at 390°F. Using cooking spray, coat a muffin pan.

⇒ In a large-sized mixing bowl, combine all of the ingredients listed above. To match your air fryer basket, cut a piece of parchment paper to fit.

⇒ Combine grated zucchini, coconut flour, grated mozzarella, black pepper, and sea salt in a large mixing bowl. Combine the melted butter and eggs.

⇒ Fill the muffin cups evenly with the zucchini mixture, packing it down the sides and smoothing the tops.

⇒ Bake for around 15 to 20 minutes, or till firm and brown on top.

⇒ Toss the muffin with a teaspoon of marinara sauce and the remaining mozzarella cheese. To taste, season with Italian spice and pepperoni slices.

Cheesy Asparagus Tots

Preparation Time: 30 minutes

Servings: 4

Nutrition Facts: Calories 78; Total Fat 3g; Carbohydrates 8g; Protein 4g

Ingredients:

o   ½ cup of panko bread crumbs

o   Cooking spray

o   ¼ cup of Parmesan cheese, grated

o   12 ounces of asparagus, trimmed and diced

Instructions:

⇒ Preheat the oven at 400°F.

⇒ On medium-high flame, bring salted water to a boil. In a pot, bring the asparagus to a boil for about 5 minutes. Drain in a colander for 5 minutes or till cold enough to handle.

⇒ In a large-sized mixing bowl, combine the asparagus, parmesan cheese, and breadcrumbs. Knead everything together with your hands till it forms a dough-like consistency. To make a tot, take one tablespoon of the mixture and roll it into a ball. Arrange the ingredients on a serving plate. Continue in the same manner with the rest of the mixture. Toasted tots should be frozen for 30 minutes.

⇒ Spray a baking sheet with nonstick cooking oil. Bake the tots for around 15 minutes.

Low-carb Tasty Crackers

Preparation Time: 25 minutes

Servings: 4

Nutrition Facts: Calories 130; Total Fat 11g; Carbohydrates 4g; Protein 6g

Ingredients:

o   1/2 cup almond flour

- o 1/2 cup cheddar cheese, shredded
- o 2 tsp paprika, divided
- o Salt
- o Water

Instructions:

⇒ Use a food processor or high-speed blender to combine almond flour, shredded cheese, and 1 tsp paprika. Blend the mixture until it forms a dough-like consistency.

⇒ If the dough is too crumbly, add a small amount of water to help bind it together.

⇒ Take the dough and place it between two sheets of parchment paper. Roll it out until it becomes flat and thin.

⇒ Use a pizza cutter to cut the flattened dough into square shapes.

⇒ Transfer the cut dough onto a baking sheet lined with parchment paper.

⇒ Bake the crackers in the oven for 10 minutes, then flip them over and continue baking for an additional 5 minutes.

⇒ Once done, remove the crackers from the oven, then season with paprika and a pinch of salt.

⇒ Allow them to cool completely before serving.

Frozen Yogurt Delight

Preparation Time: 5 minutes

Servings: 2

Nutrition Facts: Calories 128; Total Fat 1; Carbohydrates 20g; Protein 11g

Ingredients:

- o 1 cup Greek yogurt 0%
- o 1 cup frozen berries
- o 1 tbsp lemon juice, freshly squeezed
- o 1 tbsp honey
- o 3 almonds, chopped

Instructions:

⇒ In a blender, combine greek yogurt 0%, frozen berries, honey and lemon juice.

⇒ Pulse until the mixture becomes soft, and make sure not to blend too much

⇒ Divide the frozen yogurt into two cups, spread the almonds on top, and serve immediately.

Kale Chips

Preparation Time: 20 minutes

Servings: 2

Nutrition Facts: Calories 95; Total Fat 7; Carbohydrates 6g; Protein 3g

Ingredients:

o   2 cups kale leaves, stems removed
o   1 tbsp olive oil
o   1/4 tsp Himalayan salt
o   1/4 tsp black pepper

Instructions:

⇒ Preheat the oven to 300°F.

⇒ Wash the kale leaves thoroughly and dry them completely. Tear the leaves into bite-sized pieces.

⇒ In a large bowl, drizzle the kale leaves with olive oil and season with black pepper.

⇒ Toss the kale gently to ensure you coat all leaves with the oil and seasoning.

⇒ Line a baking sheet with parchment paper and place the seasoned kale leaves in a single layer.

⇒ Bake for 12 minutes or until the leaves turn crispy and slightly golden.

⇒ Remove from the oven and add Himalayan salt.

⇒ Allow them to cool completely before serving.

Avocado and Turkey Roll-Ups

Preparation Time: 10 minutes

Servings: 2

Nutrition Facts: Calories 287; Total Fat 33g; Carbohydrates 7g; Protein 36g

Ingredients:
o   1 avocado
o   8 turkey breast slices
o   2 tbsp low-fat cream cheese
o   Salt and pepper to taste
o   Optional: lemon or lime juice

Instructions:
⇒   Slice the avocado in half, remove the pit, and scoop the flesh into a bowl. Mash it with a fork, then season with salt, pepper, and any additional flavorings you prefer.
⇒   Lay the turkey slices flat on a clean surface. Spread a layer of mashed avocado onto each piece, then spread a layer of cream cheese.
⇒   Roll up the turkey slices tightly and secure them with toothpicks.
⇒   If you like it, you can drizzle the roll-ups with lemon or lime juice.
⇒   Enjoy immediately or refrigerate for later.

Tasty Roasted Chickpeas

Preparation Time: 30 minutes

Servings: 4

Nutrition Facts: Calories 160; Total Fat 9g; Carbohydrates 15g; Protein 5g

Ingredients:
- 1 can (15 ounces) chickpeas, drained and rinsed
- 2 tbsp olive oil
- 1 tsp ground cumin
- 1 tsp paprika
- 1/2 teaspoon garlic powder
- 1/2 tsp salt

Instructions:

- Preheat your oven to 400°F and line a baking sheet with parchment paper.
- Pat dry the chickpeas using a clean kitchen towel or paper towels to remove excess moisture.
- In a medium bowl, combine the chickpeas, salt, cumin, paprika, garlic powder and oil. Toss until the chickpeas are evenly coated.
- Spread the chickpeas in a single layer on the prepared baking sheet.
- Roast in the oven for 20 minutes or until golden brown and crispy, shaking the pan halfway through to ensure even cooking.
- Remove from the oven and let them cool slightly before serving. You can store them in an airtight container for a few days.

Summer Skewers

Preparation Time: 10 minutes

Servings: 2

Nutrition Facts: Calories 168; Total Fat 9g; Carbohydrates 8g; Protein 12g

Ingredients:
o 1 cup cherry tomatoes
o 1 large cucumber (cut into 1/2-inch rounds)
o 4 ounces fresh mozzarella balls (bocconcini)
o Fresh basil leaves
o Balsamic glaze
o Salt and pepper to taste
o Wooden skewers

Instructions:

⟹ Rinse the cherry tomatoes and pat them dry. Thread one cherry tomato onto each skewer, followed by a mozzarella ball, a slice of cucumber, and a fresh basil leaf.
⟹ Repeat the process until all the skewers are assembled.
⟹ Arrange the skewers on a serving platter, season with salt and pepper, and drizzle with balsamic glaze.
⟹ Serve immediately or refrigerate until ready to eat.

Healthy Zucchini Chips

Preparation Time: 30 minutes

Servings: 2

Nutrition Facts: Calories 190; Total Fat 16g; Carbohydrates 6g; Protein 5g

Ingredients:
o 2 medium zucchini
o 2 tbsp olive oil
o 1/4 cup grated Parmesan cheese
o 1/2 tsp garlic powder
o 1/2 tsp dried oregano
o Salt and pepper to taste

Instructions:
⇒ Preheat your oven to 425°F and line a baking sheet with parchment paper.
⇒ Wash the zucchini and slice them into thin rounds, about 1/8-inch thick.
⇒ In a medium bowl, toss the zucchini slices with olive oil, Parmesan cheese, garlic powder, dried oregano, salt, and pepper until well coated.
⇒ Arrange the coated zucchini slices in a single layer on the prepared baking sheet.
⇒ Bake for 15-20 minutes or until the zucchini chips are golden brown and crispy.
⇒ Remove from the oven and let them cool slightly before serving.

SMOOTHIE RECIPES

Cream Oatmeal Blueberry Smoothie

Preparation Time: 5 minutes

Servings: 4

Nutrition Facts: Calories 164; Total Fat 3g; Carbohydrates 30g; Protein 6g

Ingredients:

- 1/2 cup of low-fat Greek yogurt
- 1/2 cup of vanilla almond milk unsweetened or milk of your choice
- ½ cup of loosely packed spinach
- ¾ cup of blueberries frozen
- 1 large banana large (sliced into chunks and frozen)
- ½ cup of old fashioned rolled oats
- 1 tablespoon of ground flaxseed meal
- 2 tablespoons of honey

Instructions:

⇒ To crush the blueberries and oats, place them in the blender's base and whirl a few times. Combine the banana chunks, spinach, Greek yogurt, 2 tbsp. honey, flaxseed meal, and almond milk in a blender.

⇒ Blend until the mixture is fully smooth. Pour into jars and serve immediately.

Fruity Kale Smoothie

Preparation Time: 5 minutes

Servings: 2

Nutrition Facts: Calories 157; Total Fat 0.5g; Carbohydrates 37g; Protein 2g

Ingredients:

- 1/4 cup of plain Greek yogurt non-fat
- 3/4 cup of vanilla almond milk ,unsweetened
- 2 cups of lightly packed chopped kale leaves, remove the stems
- 1 medium banana frozen, sliced into chunks
- 1/4 cup of frozen pineapple chunks
- 2 tablespoons of crunchy or creamy peanut butter
- 1 to 2 tablespoon of honey to taste

Instructions:

⇒ In a blender, combine kale leaves, unsweetened almond milk, banana chunks, yogurt, pineapple chunks, peanut butter, and 2 tbsp. honey in the following order: kale leaves, unsweetened almond milk, banana chunks, yogurt, pineapple chunks, peanut butter, and 2 tbsp. honey

⇒ Blend until the mixture is fully smooth. Pour into jars and serve immediately.

Pineapple Chia Smoothie

Preparation Time: 5 minutes

Servings: 2

Nutrition Facts: Calories 273; Total Fat 11g; Carbohydrates 43g; Protein 5g

Ingredients:

o 1 cup of frozen pineapple chunks

o 2 medium bananas chunks

o 2 tablespoons of almond butter

o 1 tablespoon of chia seeds

o 1 cup of water

Instructions:

⇒ In a blender, combine banana pieces, pineapple chunks, almond butter, and chia seeds with water.

⇒ Blend until the mixture is fully smooth. Pour the smoothie into a glass and enjoy!

Kiwi Strawberry Smoothie

Preparation Time: 5 minutes

Servings: 2

Nutrition Facts: Calories 204; Total Fat 0.5g; Carbohydrates 45g; Protein 4.3g

Ingredients:

o 1/2 cup of skim milk

o 1/2 cup of strawberry halves frozen

o 2 ripe kiwis small, quartered, and peeled

o 1 clementine or 1/2 medium orange, peel and remove the pith

o ½ banana, sliced and frozen

o 2 tablespoons of rolled oats

o 1 tablespoon of honey, optional

o Ice cubes optional

Instructions:

⇒ In a blender, combine the ripe kiwis, strawberry halves, orange, milk, rolled oats, and ice cubes.

⇒ Blend until the mixture is fully smooth.

⇒ Taste it and then add. honey if you want to add more sweetness, then serve.

Apple, Kale, And Celery Smoothie

Preparation Time: 5 minutes

Cooking time: 0 minutes

Servings: 2

Nutrition Facts: Calories 163; Total Fat 2g; Carbohydrates 37g; Protein 3g

Ingredients

o 1 cup of kale

o 1/3 cup of flat-leaf parsley or cilantro

o 1 stalk of celery

o 1 organic apple

o   1 tablespoon of ground flaxseed

o   1/4 teaspoon of ground cinnamon

o   1 lemon, juiced

o   1 1/4 cups of chilled water

Instructions:

⇒ Combine all of the ingredients in a blender and puree until smooth. To serve, pour over ice cubes.

BONUS: 35-Day Meal Plan for Women over 50

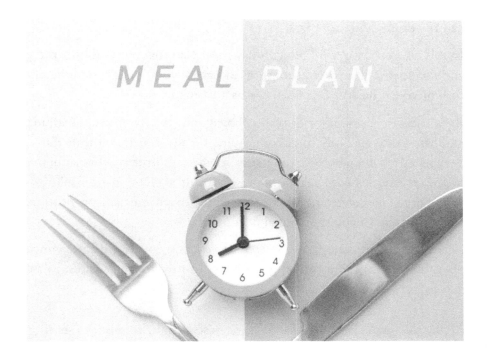

When starting with Intermittent Fasting, eating healthily during the eating time frame is essential. This is especially important if the goal is to lose weight. A balanced meal plan should include adequate calorie intake, nutrient-rich foods with a balanced ratio of macronutrients, and various foods.

It is crucial to ensure you take in enough calories during the eating windows to fuel your body and support your metabolism. You should incorporate plenty of whole, nutrient-rich foods into your meals, including lean proteins, fruits, vegetables, and healthy fats.

For maintaining energy levels and promoting satiety, a balanced intake of macronutrients (carbohydrates, proteins, and fats) is essential. With each macronutrient, aim for moderate consumption. A balanced ratio of macronutrients is approximately 45-65% of daily calories from carbohydrates, 10-35% from protein, 20-35% from fats. These ratios may vary based on individual needs and goals. For example, those following a low-carbohydrate or ketogenic diet may consume fewer carbohydrates and more fats.

In this chapter, you will find a 35-day meal plan that meets these criteria and includes a limited consumption of carbohydrates. It can be helpful for you to eat healthy and balanced as a woman over 50.

Remember to drink a lot of water throughout the day to stay hydrated and listen to your body to eat mindfully. Finally, schedule meals during designated eating windows to ensure adequate nutrition while adhering to the fasting schedule. You should consult a dietitian or healthcare professional to determine the most suitable macronutrient proportions for you based on your individual needs and goals.

I have created this shopping list to help you implement the 35-day meal plan. It includes the essential ingredients to prepare the recipes in the meal plan.

Adjust the quantities of the listed items based on the number of servings needed and your personal preferences. Consider the number of people you are cooking for, and the portion sizes required for each recipe.

Once you have all the necessary ingredients, follow the meal plan to prepare your breakfast, lunch, dinner, and snacks each day. Enjoy the variety of flavors and nutritious meals curated for you.

Remember, this shopping list serves as a guide, and you can adjust it based on your dietary preferences, allergies, and specific nutritional requirements.

Week 1

Day	Breakfast	Lunch	Dinner	Snack
1	Oat-Egg Power Breakfast	Loaded Barley Salad with Fresh Veggies	Chicken with Basil-Lemon Gravy	Almond-Garlic Crackers
2	Scrambled Egg Breakfast	Vegan Chili	Beef & Cheese Lettuce Wraps	Avocado and Turkey Roll-Ups
3	Chia Seed Banana Blueberry Delight	Zucchini Noodle Alfredo Delight	Greek-Style Feta Chicken	Tasty Roasted Chickpeas
4	Breakfast Spinach Frittata	Stuffed Zucchini Boats	Tempting Chicken Satay	Healthy Zucchini Chips
5	Blueberry and Oat Pancakes with Cinnamon	Spinach and Cheese Stuffed Mushrooms	Shrimp Skewers with Cilantro Lime	Frozen Yogurt Delight
6	Delicious Stuffed Peppers	Tempting Fish Soup	Flavorsome Almond-Crusted Tilapia	Kale Chips
7	High Protein Breakfast Cups	Cheesy Cauliflower Comfort	Dill Salmon Spiced Cumin	Almond-Garlic Crackers

Week 2

Day	Breakfast	Lunch	Dinner	Snack
8	Berry Nutty Yogurt Bowl	Cheese-Stuffed Mushrooms	Easy Beef Stew	Pizza Muffins
9	Green Toast	Vegan Chili	Beef & Cheese Lettuce Wraps	Cheesy Asparagus Tots
10	Berry Oatmeal Delight	Zucchini Noodle Alfredo Delight	Tempting Chicken Satay	Tasty Roasted Chickpeas
11	Spinach Mushroom Scramble	Stuffed Zucchini Boats	Greek-Style Feta Chicken	Frozen Yogurt Delight
12	Overnight Chia Pudding	Loaded Barley Salad with Fresh Veggies	Beef & Cheese Lettuce Wraps	Avocado and Turkey Roll-Ups
13	Oat-Egg Power Breakfast	Tempting Fish Soup	Flavorsome Almond-Crusted Tilapia	Healthy Zucchini Chips
14	Scrambled Egg Breakfast	Cheesy Cauliflower Comfort	Dill Salmon Spiced Cumin	Almond-Garlic Crackers

Week 3

Day	Breakfast	Lunch	Dinner	Snack
15	Chia Seed Banana Blueberry Delight	Stuffed Zucchini Boats	Greek-Style Feta Chicken	Tasty Roasted Chickpeas
16	Blueberry and Oat Pancakes with Cinnamon	Spinach and Cheese Stuffed Mushrooms	Shrimp Skewers with Cilantro Lime	Frozen Yogurt Delight
17	Delicious Stuffed Peppers	Tempting Fish Soup	Flavorsome Almond-Crusted Tilapia	Cheesy Asparagus Tots
18	High Protein Breakfast Cups	Cheesy Cauliflower Comfort	Beef & Cheese Lettuce Wraps	Healthy Zucchini Chips
19	Berry Nutty Yogurt Bowl	Vegan Chili	Pork Tenderloin with Leeks	Tasty Roasted Chickpeas
20	Green Toast	Loaded Barley Salad with Fresh Veggies	Dill Salmon Spiced Cumin	Almond-Garlic Crackers
21	Berry Oatmeal Delight	Zucchini Noodle Alfredo Delight	Tempting Chicken Satay	Frozen Yogurt Delight

Week 4

Day	Breakfast	Lunch	Dinner	Snack
22	Spinach Mushroom Scramble	Cheesy Cauliflower Comfort	Chicken with Basil-Lemon Gravy	Avocado and Turkey Roll-Ups
23	Overnight Chia Pudding	Stuffed Zucchini Boats	Tempting Chili Garlic Chicken	Tasty Roasted Chickpeas
24	Oat-Egg Power Breakfast	Greek-Style Feta Chicken	Shrimp Skewers with Cilantro Lime	Cheesy Asparagus Tots
25	Berry Nutty Yogurt Bowl	Loaded Barley Salad with Fresh Veggies	Flavorsome Almond-Crusted Tilapia	Healthy Zucchini Chips
26	Green Toast	Tempting Fish Soup	Pork Tenderloin with Leeks	Tasty Roasted Chickpeas
27	Berry Oatmeal Delight	Zucchini Noodle Alfredo Delight	Beef & Cheese Lettuce Wraps	Pizza Muffins
28	Delicious Stuffed Peppers	Greek-Style Feta Chicken	Dill Salmon Spiced Cumin	Frozen Yogurt Delight

Week 5

Day	Breakfast	Lunch	Dinner	Snack
29	High Protein Breakfast Cups	Cheesy Cauliflower Comfort	Chicken with Basil-Lemon Gravy	Almond-Garlic Crackers
30	Berry Nutty Yogurt Bowl	Greek-Style Feta Chicken	Shrimp Skewers with Cilantro Lime	Avocado and Turkey Roll-Ups
31	Green Toast	Tempting Fish Soup	Flavorsome Almond-Crusted Tilapia	Cheesy Asparagus Tots
32	Berry Oatmeal Delight	Loaded Barley Salad with Fresh Veggies	Pork Tenderloin with Leeks	Healthy Zucchini Chips
33	Spinach Mushroom Scramble	Stuffed Zucchini Boats	Tempting Chili Garlic Chicken	Tasty Roasted Chickpeas
34	Overnight Chia Pudding	Vegan Chili	Beef & Cheese Lettuce Wraps	Pizza Muffins
35	Oat-Egg Power Breakfast	Zucchini Noodle Alfredo Delight	Dill Salmon Spiced Cumin	Frozen Yogurt Delight

Shopping list

Category	Items
PROTEINS	Eggs, Chicken breasts, Tuna, Shrimp, Tilapia fillets, Salmon fillets, Ground beef, Pork tenderloin, Feta cheese, Cheddar cheese, Ground turkey
FRUITS	Bananas, Blueberries, Strawberries, Kiwi, Apples, Pineapple
VEGETABLES	Spinach, Mushrooms, Peppers (bell peppers and jalapenos), Leeks, Asparagus, Kale, Zucchini, Cauliflower, Celery
GRAINS AND LEGUMES	Oats, Barley, Chia seeds, Almond flour, Cumin, Chickpeas, Whole grain bread, Tortillas
DAIRY AND DAIRY ALTERNATIVES	Greek yogurt, Plant-based yogurt, Low-fat cheese, Almond milk or other plant-based milk
PANTRY STAPLES	Olive oil, Garlic, Onion, Chili garlic sauce, Cilantro, Dijon mustard, Vegetable broth, Tomato sauce, Red pepper flakes, Paprika, Salt, Pepper
SNACKS	Almonds, Whole grain crackers, Frozen yogurt, Kale chips, Avocado, Turkey slices, Roasted chickpeas, Skewers, Zucchini chips
SMOOTHIE INGREDIENTS	Rolled oats, Almond milk or other plant-based milk, Protein powder, Nut butter, Greek yogurt or plant-based yogurt, Honey or other sweetener

Conclusion

By the end of this book, I hope you've gained some valuable insights into intermittent fasting for women over 50. We've covered a lot of ground together, diving into the science behind fasting, exploring different protocols, and giving you practical tips to kick-start your fasting journey.

I won't sugarcoat it—switching to intermittent fasting can be challenging. It takes dedication, perseverance, and a willingness to challenge old beliefs and habits. But let me tell you, the rewards are so worth it! Intermittent fasting goes way beyond just shedding some pounds. It's a powerful tool that can transform your health, boost your energy levels, and reshape your entire relationship with food.

As a woman over 50, you can embrace your body, take control of your well-being, and feel vibrant and alive. Throughout this book, we've busted myths, tackled common challenges, and even shared mouthwatering recipes to support you. Armed with knowledge and practical tools, you're now ready to embark on this transformative journey with confidence and grace.

Now, here's a little reminder for you: your journey is YOURS. Listen to your body, honor its needs, and don't be afraid to make adjustments along the way. Be kind to yourself, have patience, and celebrate every step forward, no matter how small. And hey, if you're looking for extra support, consider joining online groups or using apps specifically designed for intermittent fasting—they can be real game-changers!

Oh, and I've got something special for you—a 35-day meal plan and a shopping list to help you kick-start your fasting journey. But don't feel limited by it. Feel free to get creative, try new things, and make this fasting lifestyle truly your own.

Stay connected with your body, mind, and spirit as you continue on this path. Keep that initial spark alive and envision the vibrant, healthy, and empowered version of yourself that you're becoming. Surround yourself with a supportive community, seek guidance when needed, and celebrate each and every victory, big or small.

Now, if you've enjoyed this book and found it helpful, I would be thrilled if you could take a moment to share your honest thoughts and experiences by leaving a review on Amazon. Your feedback is not only invaluable for other readers, but it also fuels my motivation to keep creating content that supports and inspires women on their intermittent fasting journey.

Thank you from the bottom of my heart for joining me on this inspiring and life-changing adventure. I'm truly grateful to have been a part of your journey.

With gratitude,

Mary K. Day

Made in the USA
Las Vegas, NV
18 October 2023

79274901R00059